Eat
SLENDER

Do NOT let your *wayward hormones* make you fat!

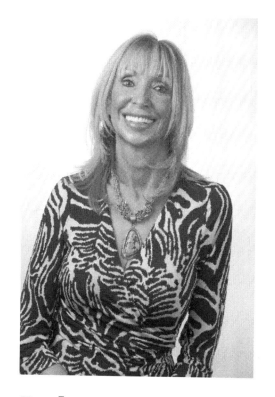

Barbara A. Hoffman

Imagine the day when you can
truly EAT and lose weight
That day is here!

Eat Yourself
SLENDER

By Barbara A. Hoffman

This book is intended as a reference volume only, not as a medical manual. The information given here is designed to help you make informed decisions about your health. The dietary programs in this book are not intended as a substitute for any dietary regimen that may have been prescribed by your doctor. If you have a medical condition you should discuss all new dietary programs with your doctor before beginning.

First Edition: September, 2012. Printed in the USA. International Standard Book Number: 978-0-9753353-0-7

Cover photo: Tony Florez Photography

Cover page & design: Jessica Prussa & Nicole Pillsbury

Editor: Erica Wang

Trademarks
All terms mentioned in this book that are known to be trademarks or service marks have been appropriately capitalized. Trademarks belong to the appropriate companies.

About The Author

Barbara A. Hoffman

Barbara Hoffman is a Naturopath, medical researcher & journalist, women's health advocate and natural hormone and weight consultant. She is also a television producer and for 11 years, she produced a cable network television program which focused on health and wellness.

Barbara has been in the medical field for over 30 years and worked in the field of women's health since 1980. For the past 20 years she has been researching weight loss, the benefits of natural progesterone, writing about alternatives to synthetic hormones, and compiling weight loss studies.

Her passion to teach fuels her mission to empower women to make more educated and informed choices about their health.

Barbara resides in Orange County, California. She has been married for 26 years and has one son.

Dedication

I want to thank some very special people who have donated many hours of their precious time helping me to bring this book to print. Thank you, Jessica Prussa, Nicole Pillsbury and Erica Wang for your diligence, organizational and editing skills and your always uplifting faith in me. I so appreciate your faithful hearts and encouragement. You have truly been "God's hands extended to me on this Earth. I hope that I serve you as well as you have served me.

Thank you to my beloved husband, David, who cheerfully "ate himself slender" all the while pushing me towards my greatest good.

I extend my heartfelt thank you and admiration to the Daystar Television Network. Daystar is an abiding source of spiritual guidance in my daily life for which I am deeply grateful. Immersion in God's word and God's people helps me to sing a new song every day.

Most of all, thank you Holy Spirit for your presence and wisdom and for filling me with the utmost desire to help God's wonderful people live long and healthy lives.

More special thanks go to all of the marvelous people who have called, written, emailed and texted me their thoughts, tips and encouragement. You are the reason I write and will continue to write so that you can have "Better Health Naturally."

One more acknowledgment: my 22-year old son, Drew Christian. At 16, he wisely discharged me as a "helicopter Mom" which freed me up to become the weight watchdog for all of you who are reading this book. I truly care about you all!

Introduction

The Secret of Weight Loss

Dear Friends:

Do you want to eat AND lose weight?
It's much easier than you think!

I have been interested in weight loss since I was 22
years old and a "boyfriend" called me "chunky". Believe
me, he was no friend. I embarked on a series of brutal
dieting for the next 8 years. I tried high protein, counting
carbs, eliminating fat, the cabbage soup diet, the Stillman
diet, the Atkins diet and even taken diet pills. Guess
what? I did lose weight, but I was always miserable,
tired, and hungry and I lost my JOY! Then I would just
gain all the weight back. Now, many years later after
much research, I have the answer to losing and
maintaining.

Let this book be your guide to my weight loss and weight
maintenance program. I've helped many men and
women just like you. Now it's YOUR turn to "Eat Yourself
Slender".

Read on to find the answer to why dieting does not work
(you already knew this) and why eating does work. You
were designed by God to eat good foods.
This plan will change your life!

Your friend for Better Health,
Barbara A. Hoffman.

Eat Yourself
SLENDER

Table of Contents

Guess What?
EATING LESS DOES NOT WORK
EXERCISING MORE DOES NOT WORK!
TASTELESS HEALTH FOODS DO NOT WORK
UNHEALTHY CLEANSES DO NOT WORK

The **3 keys to successful weight loss** are:

1. SUGAR IS YOUR ENEMY
2. PROTEIN IS YOUR FRIEND
3. YOUR BRAIN NEURONS MUST BE NOURISHED AND IN BALANCE

HERE IS WHAT ELSE I CAN TELL YOU:
1) Counting calories absolutely does not work
2) You DO NOT have to spend all your time at a gym
3) You can eat! You can eat yourself slender!

Your strategy is NOT going to be:
Have a salad and take a walk. No, no, no! You are going to EAT! You do NOT have to be hungry.
We are NOT going to change your calories, just your carbohydrate intake

THE MECHANISM
Foods can either:
   1) **Cause fat burning**
   2) **Cause fat storage**

If you chronically elevate your blood sugar with carbohydrates and sugar, your body has no choice but to release insulin to take care of the sugar.
The fat cells of adipose tissue are extremely sensitive to insulin compared to other tissues in the body.
Too much insulin tells your body to store fat!

150 years of anecdotal evidence shows us that carbs and starch make us fat. Our mothers knew this! They served us protein and vegetables.

CARBOHYDRATES DRIVE INSULIN, INSULIN DRIVES FAT.

It's not about calories!
Why are so many poor people fat? Think about it. They don't eat out in restaurants. They don't have a lot of food and many of them perform manual labor. So it is not "calories in, calories out" that determines weight gain or weight loss.

We don't get fat because we over-eat. We over-eat because we have excess fat. Fat cells determine how hungry you are and how much energy you will expend. The fat cells are regulated by insulin.

Under-eating does NOT cure obesity. Just about every overweight person has tried it...IT DOES NOT WORK! Even just by eating 800-1000 calories per day, only 1 in 20 patients lost any significant weight according to a large research study. Over 800 obese and overweight people were enrolled and were instructed to eat 750 calories less per day. They were also given intense counseling to help them stay on track and also given a lot of help with meal plans that were low in calories. The average participant was 50 pounds over weight. Despite all this diligence and denial, they only lost only 9 pounds in 6 months! AND they gained it back after a year. **Overeating is not the cause of all obesity and under-eating is not the cure.**

You can gain weight & grow obese on a diet of celery and vegetables, a calorie intake inadequate for even a child. I KNOW you have all tried that at one time. I certainly did, I was miserable.

In 2011 an Australian study was released that will shock you! Subjects that were on a strict low calorie diet for one year lost just short of 30 pounds. But for at least a year after the low-calorie diet, the people reported that they were significantly hungrier than they had been BEFORE THE DIETS. This is because the hormones of hunger rebounded with a vengeance and sent a single message to the person: EAT MORE! They rapidly regained the weight. Imagine being stringent and deprived for an entire year and then spending another entire year being *hungrier than ever before.*

Perhaps the best study I have seen was published in the Journal of the American Medical Association in 2007. It was called the A to Z Weight Loss Study and compared 4 diets. These were all **low carbohydrate** diets. They all worked!

The Bottom Line:
- When insulin levels drop, fat escapes from cells, fat deposits shrink
- When insulin is chronically elevated, fat accumulates in fat tissue

You want to be in fat-burning mode, not fat-storage mode. It's really simple! I will show you how.

In the past year I have helped many men & women lose weight while retaining their sense of balance and JOY! My husband lost 37 pounds in about 6 months and feels WONDERFUL!

So…my dear friends, here is the plan for you.
This is your new fun way to be healthy, slender and FULL! No more deprivation. No more hunger! No more diets!
You will be slender and you will have energy and feel great. You can eat out in restaurants, enjoy wonderful lunches and dinners and not gain another unwanted pound.
Whether you want to lose 10 pounds or 100 pounds, the process is the same. AND, it can be fun!
I am here to help you every step of the way!

Both men and women have lost 10-15 pounds the first month and ARE ABLE TO MAINTAIN THE WEIGHT LOSS. You may lose weight slower and that's fine. You will not have feelings of denial and feelings of being overwhelmed with constantly thinking about dieting.

You DO NOT have to be hungry all the time to lose weight. Low carbs are the key. **Low carb eaters give less thought to forbidden foods and are not always hungry**. Also, with sufficient protein, lean muscle mass will increase & clothing sizes are often reduced. If you cut carbs & eat more protein and fat, you won't eat if you're not hungry, just as you won't drink water if you are not thirsty, even though it's there.

**"Obesity is a disorder of fat accumulation not a disorder of over-eating".
Gary Faubes, author of Good Calories, Bad Calories**

Repeat after me:

"I am not stuck with this extra weight!"

It doesn't matter if you are busy, eat out a lot, travel or don't exercise because you don't have the time. This will work for you. Just give me 21 days, stick with it and I guarantee you will lose weight.

Second, I'm going to teach you how to eliminate cravings, binge eating, and eating the wrong foods. To do this, you are going to cut out trigger foods.
What are these?

They are **high carbohydrate foods** such as ice cream, chocolate, fried goods of any sort, chips, and cookies. You know what **YOUR** trigger is.

Wouldn't it be great NOT to crave it anymore?

Do you have that little voice in your head telling you:
- "Keep eating" (even when you know you have had enough)
- "You need something sugary, NOW."
- "Hurry up, eat that bread. You know you're hungry and can't wait for your entrée."

THIS WILL STOP!

HOW LONG WILL IT BE BEFORE I SEE RESULTS?

You should start to feel more in control of your eating very rapidly. People report losing cravings in the first week or so. Sluggish metabolism often speeds up, especially with the use of supplements and progesterone creme. You will find that you think less and less about "living to eat" and more about "eating to live." Your eating life becomes joyful and easy. Weight loss will begin within the first 2 weeks and should be steady. Mood changes are almost *immediate.*

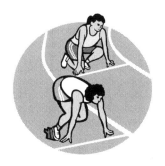

YAY! Let's get started!

Chapter 1

What Am I Doing Wrong?

Does this sound familiar?

Breakfast
Black coffee
1/2 grapefruit

Lunch
Scoop of tuna or cottage cheese or small salad

Dinner
Small piece of chicken or meat
Steamed veggies
1/2 baked potato

Snacks
Saltine crackers
Fruit

YOU ARE COUNTING CALORIES. STOP IT!
You will be miserable and you will not sustain any weight that you do lose.

WHAT'S WRONG WITH LOW CALORIE DIETS?
These starve the body of protein that is required for energy. Your fatty tissue is not targeted. **In fact, your fat cells will work overtime to hang on to their fat.** Your body will also reduce its energy production and "slow down" If you are cutting all calories across the board, you will still be eating a disproportionate amount of carbs which will still impede any lasting weight loss.

> **Eliminate STARCH, FLOUR, WHITE SUGAR and INCREASE PROTEIN and you WILL lose weight.**
> **I PROMISE**

THE OLD FOOD PYRAMID WAS WRONG!

The government was pushing us to eat less fat and more carbohydrates. NO, WRONG, WRONG!

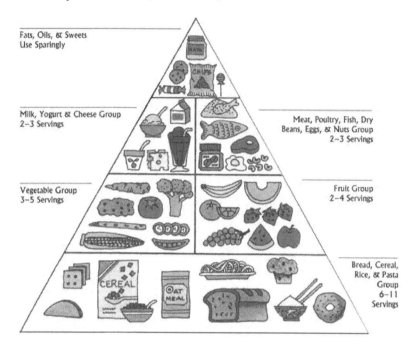

Take a look....no wonder we all got fat. It includes sugary foods on the bottom rung! Finally it got revised in **2011** but even now there are too many carbs. A government health official was interviewed on a talk show and said "we have to meet people where they are at" Imagine that! Meet us at "fat" and we will stay fat. Fifty years after the original food pyramid was given to us, we are the heaviest people on the planet.

According to this pyramid, you could have No butter, No sour cream, but it was okay to eat potatoes and white starches, up to 6 – 11 servings per day of pasta, potatoes, rice, and bread.

The healthy diet became a **low fat** diet. Where were the good fats and proteins?
Surprise! Obesity began rising at an alarming rate.

On low fat:
- Weights went up
- Portion sizes went up
- The amount of food people ate went up
- Statistics show that we are going to die younger than our parents who ate fat and protein and very little junk food.
- Over past 25 years. Americans have become heavier and diabetes has become rampart.
- By 2004, 1 in 3 American were obese
- 2 in 3 were over weight
- 1 in 10 had type II diabetes

Fat is necessary. Our brain is 70% fat, mostly in the form of myelin, which covers our nerve cells. The brain needs fat.
Also, consider the "French Paradox": People in France consume lots of saturated fat, but have comparatively little heart disease. Fat is not the demon food.

SIMPLE CARBS ARE THE CULPRIT
Fact: Obese people favor carbohydrates. They do not appear to eat more calories than lean people, they **eat more carbs**.

You chronically elevate insulin levels when you eat carbs. This causes chronic accumulation of fat in your fat tissue which becomes very difficult to lose.

Study: In the 1960's at UCLA obese patients were put on a starvation fast of periods of 12 – 117 days.
When protein & fat were added back in, patients still felt no hunger. When **carbs** were added, patients were overwhelmed with hunger and suffered all the symptoms of food deprivation.

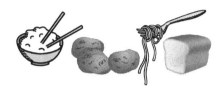

"There is something about carbohydrates that allows the consumption of enormous quantities of food (up to 2000 calories) and yet still induces hunger as night approaches". From Good Calories, Bad Calories. Gary Taubes, 2007

Your Brain on Carbs = CRAVINGS Ouch!
High-carb diets cause neurotransmitter imbalances that lead to food cravings. You will crave sugary snacks and caffeine, which will only temporarily make you feel better. The cravings can be uncontrollable and ultimately you give in.

Result: The fat builds up in the abdominal area

You MUST avoid low fat, high carb eating because it:
It adds body fat
Worsens insulin resistance
Worsens adrenal exhaustion

Chapter 2

The Plan Overview

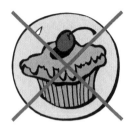

1. Sugar is the Enemy: It is toxic beyond its calories

SUGAR IS NOT YOUR FRIEND and it is very ADDICTIVE

Sugar will turn into FAT in your body, raise your cholesterol and raise your triglycerides.

CARBS TURN TO SUGAR when you eat them. Yes, that's right! S-U-G-A-R. All carbs will do this, some more slowly than others. Complex carbs found in bread, grains are slower BUT STILL TURN TO SUGAR, simple carbs such as those found in refined sugar turn quickly, fructose from fruit also turns to sugar, as do the carbs in starches like rice and pasta.

If you chronically eat too many carbs, you will become insulin resistant, which will make you even FATTER.

You have to give up sugar and carbs so your body will START TO BURN FAT. It will seek the glucose it needs in the fat storage areas.

Then you will see yourself start to lose the weight!

Please try it for 2 weeks and see how good you will feel in addition to losing pounds!

SHOCKER:

Four grams of sugar in a product = 1 Level teaspoons of white sugar

A lunch that contains 40 grams of sugar is equivalent to eating 10 TEASPOONS OF SUGAR. Most fast food meals will contain this much sugar. You might as well just pull out the sugar bowl and eat directly out of it.

Your body will not be able to burn all this sugar and it will get stored as FAT. As your insulin levels rise you will be hungrier and hungrier and crave more sugary foods.

SUGAR IS EVERYWHERE. START READING YOUR LABELS

See Chapter 17 for the Sugar Challenge!

When you first try to give up sugar, it will almost be painful if your body is addicted. You will crave it! There are some really good supplements we can discuss that will help with this. See Chapter 11

Nutrition Facts
Serving Size 8 fl oz (240ml)
Servings Per Container 1

Amount Per Serving	
Calories 110	Calories from Fat 0

	% Daily Value
Total Fat 0g	0%
Sodium 0mg	0%
Potassium 450mg	13%
Total Carbohydrate 26g	9%
Sugars 22g	
Protein 2g	

Vitamin C	120%	Calcium	2%
Thiamin	10%	Riboflavin	4%
Niacin	4%	Vitamin B6	6%
Folate	15%	Magnesium	6%

*Percent Daily Values are based on a 2,000 calorie diet. Your daily values may be higher or lower depending on your calorie needs.

Ingredients: 100% pure Florida squeezed orange juice

2. FAT-FREE IS NOT GOOD!
The food manufacturers simply substitute sugar for the fat to restore some of the taste.

3. BE CAREFUL WITH FRUIT

Fruit contains fructose which, believe it or not, can be fattening. I know many menopausal women in particular who will gain weight the day after they eat too much fruit. I tested it on myself and a day after I ate nectarines and melon and a pear (all good, right?) I gained 1.5 pounds. WOW! Who knew? So be careful with fruit. Think about it....fruit used to be seasonal and our ancestors just ate what was in season. Now we have so much available that we eat all fruits all the time. For myself, upon experimenting, I have found that I am okay with blueberries, cherries, and apples YAY! Do your own experiment to find your good fruits that will not store as fat.

Note: 1 cup of grapes will turn into about 6 teaspoons of sugar in your body. A banana? 4 teaspoons. The lowest amount of sugar is found in oranges, peaches, and berries.

4. EAT A PROTEIN BREAKFAST

Are you eating toast for breakfast? Please stop! The usual 2 slices of toast converts to about 6 teaspoons of sugar! No more cereal, bagels, or even oatmeal in most cases unless you are putting protein powder in it. For most commercial cereals, you would do better if you threw away the cereal and ate the box!

Change Your Breakfast! This one simple step can change your weight and your life.

5. NO DAIRY EXCEPT YOGURT & CREAM FOR YOUR COFFEE

- Milk raises insulin levels
- Elimination of dairy accelerates weight loss

6. LEGUMES ARE YOUR NEW BEST FRIEND

- Canned beans & lentils are fine. Rinse & drain.
- Experiment with red, black, pinto, etc.
- Add spices/ vinegar/ hot sauce
- Make fake mashed potatoes. Put a little olive oil in a pan. Heat.

Add a can of white kidney beans & mash with a spoon. You can add some water to get the desired consistency. Add salt, pepper, garlic powder, even butter and parmesan cheese. Tastes GREAT! You can also do this with steamed cauliflower. Yummy!

Tip: Mix lentils or beans with some steamed veggies and salsa. Top with some protein like chicken or left-over beef, you can even add avocado. This tastes like a burrito without the tortilla. Delicious!

7. AVOCADOS ARE GOOD FOR YOU!

- 60% more potassium than bananas
- Prevent stroke
- Lower cholesterol
- Contain 75% insoluble fiber

THE 9 SIMPLE RULES TO
EATING YOURSELF SLENDER:

1) **Avoid White Carbohydrates.**
   The Whiter the Food, The Fatter You Will Get
   "The more bread, the sooner dead."
   Specifically:
   - Bread
   - Rice
   - Cereal
   - Potatoes
   - Pasta
   - Tortillas
   - Any breaded fried foods

2) **START YOUR DAY WITH PROTEIN – every day!** Protein, protein, protein. It is almost impossible to overeat protein, so don't worry.

The Good News About Protein:
Protein improves insulin levels.
Protein is usually burned for energy and NOT stored as fat as carbs are. Protein curbs hunger so you do not overeat and snack too much between meals. Protein takes longer to break down in your body and keeps you satisfied longer. Researchers in France found that high-carb snackers got hungry JUST AS QUICKLY as people who had NO SNACKS AT ALL. Those who snacked on chicken (protein) stayed full almost 40 minutes longer. Now, that is significant!

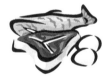

YOU NEED PROTEIN WITH EVERY MEAL!

Protein causes the brain to produce dopamine, which gives you energy and focus. Protein also helps boost your metabolism. A study from Purdue University showed that people who ate 30% of their calories from protein lost more weight than those who ate only 18%. Protein is important!

3) Eat Repetitiously

Eat the same meals over and over. There are about 50,000 products in an average grocery store. Most will make you fat.

Pick 5 meals and repeat them. If you eat out, substitute a salad or veggies in place of potatoes or rice. Tell the waiter you are on a Special Diet. You are! The "I won't be fat a minute longer diet". By the way, the true definition of diet comes from the Greek word "diaita" meaning lifestyle, NOT deprivation!

4) Eat 4 times per day

- Breakfast
- Lunch
- Afternoon smaller lunch. Calling this "lunch" will help you avoid snack foods
- Dinner

5) Never Drink Your Calories

    a. No fruit juice
    b. No soy milk
    c. No soft drinks

Drink: tea, coffee, sparkling water and water

6) **Be careful with fruit.** Fructose is a simple sugar.

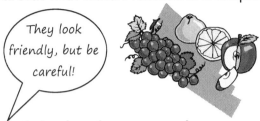

They look friendly, but be careful!

7) **Take a 1 day break every week**
Mine is Sunday. Eat whatever you want on this day. After a few weeks you will find you don't want to eat unhealthy on your "day off".

8) **NO LOW-FAT DIETING!**
When you eat a low-fat diet, your intake of carbs increases, causing high levels of sugar. This excess sugar is converted to triglycerides and is stored as FAT. Years of a low fat diet results in shrinking of muscle mass, less dense bones, increased blood pressure, increased cholesterol and WEIGHT GAIN. You need fats, you do NOT need sugar.

9) **NEVER LET YOURSELF GET TOO HUNGRY**
When you EYSS you will NOT be hungry! If you do feel hungry, you did not eat enough for your breakfast, lunch or dinner.
So eat some more! But no sugar or starch.
You will not gain weight. Right now as I am writing, I feel hungry and it is just 2 pm. I am fixing myself a hard boiled egg (GREAT snacks, so keep on hand) and I mixed it with some Thousand Island Dressing, some lemon pepper and smushed it up in a little bowl. Yummy and so filling. It will all burn off and not be stored! There are other snack tips in Chapter 9.

NOTES:

Chapter 3
Sugar Is Your Enemy.
Getting off is Step 1.

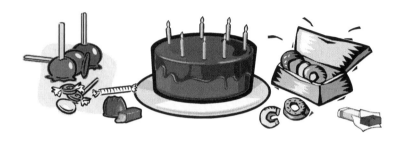

Okay, lay your cards on the table.
Are YOU addicted to Sugar?
Do you suspect that you are?

We can BREAK that addiction. I promise you! We will do
it in a series of steps that will NOT be painful.
Sugar addiction can be just as powerful as addiction to
drugs like heroin or cocaine. Once the body starts
craving it, the cravings demand to be fed. The result of
sugar addiction is obesity, diabetes, heart disease,
cancer, loss of brain function, hormone imbalance,
premature aging and depression and/or anxiety.

SUGAR IS MORE A DRUG THAN A FOOD!
(Sugar Addiction is actually an eating disorder)
That is why you have to detox from it! Researchers have
discovered that sugar and its substitutes *can surpass
the reward feeling associated with cocaine use!*

HOW DO I KNOW IF I AM TRULY ADDICTED?

- I feel moody if I don't eat sugar
- The smell or sight of sugary foods gives me a high or a "rushy" feeling and I begin craving the food
- When I am not eating sugar, I am thinking about it
- I cannot go one day without sugar
- I crave something sweet after every meal
- I crave sweets in the middle of the afternoon
- I have sugar in my coffee or tea, more than I know I should
- I start my day with something sweet like cereal, pastry or a muffin
- When I do eat sugary foods, I have no impulse control or portion control and I will eat too much

It is not just that a chocolate chip cookie tastes good to you and you would like to have one. Instead, your body absolutely cries out for that cookie to the point of anxiety and compulsion. You have activated your addiction, akin to an alcoholic and his alcohol. It is not because you have weak willpower, but that the "drug" of sugar has captured you. Sugar becomes a trigger; when you eat some you cannot stop.

DID YOU KNOW?

- Sugar Addiction is a sign of a brain neurotransmitter deficiency of serotonin and/or dopamine. They are responsible for our search for rewarding foods.
- According to Dr. Robert Rakowski, neurotransmitter imbalances can be passed down to the 4th generation! So you are not just stopping your own addiction but possibly those of your children and grandchildren.

Have you noticed, each generation seems to be getting worse with their eating habits? Stop the cycle!

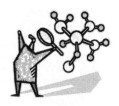

HERE IS ABSOLUTELY COMPELLING RESEARCH:

At Princeton University, internationally famous neuroscientist Dr. Bartley G. Hoebel has spent 40 years studying appetite and addictive behavior. Using laboratory rats, Dr. Hoebel gave them a 10% sugar and water solution. He was shocked when after **just a few days** the rats became addicted to the sugar solution. He says "The rats would run to the front of the cage and try to get the sugar. Sometimes, when I stuck the nozzle of the sugar-water bottle in front of the cage, they got so excited that they'd rip the stopper right off the bottle.." He found that when the rats got food and sugar water at the same time, they would turn away from the food to slurp the sugar water. When the sugar was taken away, the rats would experience severe withdrawal symptoms including shakes and chattering teeth as if they were de-toxing from a drug high. They would even walk across an electric floor that was giving them shocks in order to get to sugar water!
Do you want this *drug* controlling YOUR body?

It's Getting Worse

Guess what? McDonalds corporation is hot on the trail of sugar addicts. In November, 2011 the restaurant chain launched a plan to transform itself into a "dessert destination" because, it says, "that is what customers want" (reported in the Wall Street Journal).

McDonalds will add shakes topped with whipped crème and a cherry, strawberry crème pie with a sugar cookie crust and sugar glaze, a S'More pie, and a chocolate dipped ice cream cone. McDonalds knows that customers will buy and eat these new sugar concoctions because their statistics reveal that 20% of their existing apple pies are sold at breakfast alone!

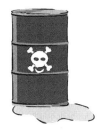

<u>High Fructose Corn Syrup is Almost a Poison</u>

In the 1970s, something awful happened to us: corn sweetener. The sugar blends in corn syrup (called dextrose, dextrin, fructose, and/or high fructose corn syrup) are actually a class of chemicals. You may mistakenly believe that it comes from fruit because of the word "fructose". It does not; it is a starch and it does NOT EXIST IN NATURE!
High fructose corn syrup (HFCS) is ubiquitous today.

Here is what it does to your body:
- Raises cholesterol and low-density lipoproteins (LDL) in your bloodstream
- Significantly raises triglyceride levels in the bloodstream
- Creates WRINKLES!! Your cellular metabolism breaks down and collagen is DAMAGED.

Your brain does not recognize HFCS as sugar. Therefore you do not get the signal to stop eating it. THIS IS THE WORST FORM OF SUGAR. It will actually age your cells!

Why has this fake sugar been foisted on us?

HFCS is:
- Cheaper. Sugar costs around 30 cents per pound;
- 10 Cents per pound. That's why a "Super Size" drink is so cheap.
- Easier to process, has a long shelf life, keeps baked goods soft and gives food a nice brown toasted color.

IT SOUNDS GOOD, BUT IT IS ESSENTIALLY POISON TO YOUR SYSTEM!

HELP ME! HOW DO I GET OFF SUGAR?
You will slowly decrease the amount of sugar you are using. We will take it one step at a time.

We will balance your brain's chemistry to beat the feelings of sugar withdrawal.

You can notice the difference in as little as 1 week! Over time, you will beat the addiction entirely.

I DID IT AND I WANT TO HELP YOU.
IT FEELS FANTASTIC!

Why Do I Have A Sweet Tooth Anyway?

God gave us a sweet tooth for a reason. Humans c
make our own Vitamin C as animals do. Vitamin C i
found mostly in fruits and God gave us taste buds th
make these sweeter-tasting foods desirable so we would
get Vitamin C from them. End of story? No, of course not!
Man got involved and started adding sugar to so many
other products and our taste buds began to crave those
products. God did not intend for you to crave a Dunkin
Donut.
An orange, yes!

How much sugar can I eat if I want to Eat Myself Slender?

THE ANSWER IS: **NOT MUCH!**

For healthy people, about 2 teaspoons of added sugar at
one time about twice a day is enough for your body to
handle. If you have any health issues, I believe your body
is not truly equipped to handle any sugar!
Start reading labels today! Take the grams of sugar for
each serving and divide by 4. That equals one teaspoon
of sugar!

If a carton of yogurt contains 12 grams of sugar, that is 3
teaspoons of sugar. Imagine sitting and eating 3
teaspoons of white sugar for your breakfast or lunch or
snack. No wonder we are feeling tired, anxious,
depressed or just plain awful! WATCH THOSE LABELS!
Make a game out of it and just REFUSE to purchase
those foods or to eat them. Your health is your wealth.
Do NOT give it up to sugar!

THE DEADLY TRIO: SUGAR-FAT-SALT
IT'S OUT TO GET YOU!

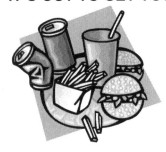

This is a DEADLY, ADDICTIVE combination! Combining Sugar/Fat/Salt intentionally increases the hedonic value of food (gives immediate pleasure). The sweeter, the saltier, the fattier the food, the more your neurons are stimulated. This prompts a strong emotional response. Your body begins to desire reaching its "Bliss Point" and wants MORE & MORE.

The fast food industry knows the addictive properties of SUGAR-FAT-SALT and incorporates it into their foods. They want you to return again and again! Prime examples are a crispy food with a salty and sweet taste (chicken nuggets) or a fatty food with a sweet taste (milk shakes). Chicken nuggets are loaded with salt and fat. Then sugar is mixed into the fat. Also, did you know that even the fast food hamburger buns have sugar in them? Yes! Furthermore, the beef patties can have sugar added as a flavor enhancer.

French fries: just potatoes right? No! Fast food french fries are frequently dipped in a sugar solution before frying. Yikes! The potato breaks down to sugar in your body. When you add ketchup, you add even more sugar!

The S-S-F combination temporarily increases dopamine in the brain and then **just leaves you wanting more!**

The S-S-F combination also breaks down in the mouth in an unhealthy manner. The small round mass of chewed food is called a bolus. The bolus of sugary foods feels slippery, soft, and juicy very fast. The body does not need to chew much and thus does not begin to feel satiated so you want more! This is done intentionally by the fast food industry. They are layering sugar onto fat onto salt and selling it to us and our children to get us addicted.

The addiction can get to the point whereby you can drive past a specific location and begin salivating for a specific food that you remember eating. Your body/brain begins incessantly nudging you to stop and GET THAT FOOD; that highly palatable food. Even a billboard can stimulate some people into impulsive behavior. You become anxious, preoccupied and have to satisfy the urge. Coffee shops have also gotten into the act. Do you crave a regular cup of coffee? Sometimes, but 90% of the time it is the Frappacino that you crave. This is S-S-F loaded into coffee! Sugary flavors are manipulated to keep you wanting more and coming back.

We are making ourselves and our children sick! Babies like a sweet taste. Once they become addicted to the taste, they will go back for more and more.

Children are getting high blood pressure between the ages of 8 – 17!
Cholesterol is high in 5th graders now!
Adolescents are developing stomach cancer.
Since the 1980's the chance of a young adult getting stomach cancer has increased by 70%

What has Sugar-Fat-Salt Done to our Weight?
In 1960 the average 40 year old woman weighed 142 pounds. In 2000 she weighs 169 pounds.
This is frightening! What has changed?
Fast food became ubiquitous in America.
A single meal from a fast food restaurant can contain your entire calorie quota for one day, not to mention the hidden sugars! DO NOT FALL INTO THE TRAP!

If you are having any difficulty, I sincerely hope you are reaching out for the support you need. I truly enjoy hearing from you and being your cheerleader as we go forth, so do not hesitate to call me! My husband is now celebrating
one year without sugar and he looks and feels like a new man. I am into my 5th year and when I celebrated my birthday this year, I felt like the clock was turning back, not ahead!
My mood and energy and weight are completely stable and I feel fantastic! As a former carb / sugar-a-holic, I want this for you!

HOW WILL I FEEL WHEN I CUT OUT SUGAR?

At first YOU may feel moody or irritable. This will pass in 7-10 days. To ease yourself through this, eat THE BEST DARK CHOCOLATE YOU CAN FIND!
Really dark chocolate has no milk and less sugar. It does not breakdown collagen and elastic tissue like sugary chocolate does. If you are craving a sweet, go for dark chocolate-covered almonds. Those are the best!

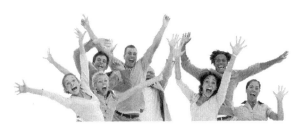

Finally, the Jack LaLanne story.

Let THIS be your inspiration!

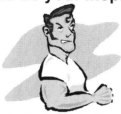

LaLanne's father died of a heart attack at age 50. His mother began to spoil him, giving him sweets as a reward. By the time he reached adolescence he had become a "sugarholic" with a violent temper and suicidal thoughts. But that was only the beginning: He was failing in school, his stomach was upset, he wore glasses, he had terrible headaches, he was weak and skinny, and he had pimples and boils.

"I was demented! I was psychotic! It was like a horror movie!" LaLanne said of this time of his life.

When he was 15, his distressed mother dragged him to a lecture on healthful living being given by nutritionist Paul Bragg. At some point Bragg asked the young LaLanne what he had eaten for breakfast, lunch and dinner, and Jack replied: "Cakes, pies and ice cream!" He said, "Jack, you are a walking garbage can." But Bragg offered nutritional salvation to Lalanne. He could be "born again" and be the healthful and strong person he wanted to be - if he changed his ways.

Lalanne took Bragg's message fully to heart. By his own testimony and that of everyone around him, he never had cake, pie, ice cream or any sweet <u>from that day forward</u>. All his maladies disappeared; he even stopped wearing glasses. "I was a whole new human being," he said of this transformation. "I liked people, they liked me. It was like an exorcism, kicking the devil outta me!"

THIS CAN BE YOU!

Chapter 4

Why am I fat, I don't eat a lot? Insulin Is the Culprit

WHAT IS INSULIN?

Most people never worry about insulin unless they have diabetes. But guess what?

INSULIN IS THE FAT STORAGE HORMONE and will make you FAT! When you eat carbs you raise your blood sugar and stimulate the release of insulin. Insulin tells the body to store the sugar (glucose) for future use. The body also creates glycogen, strings of glucose molecules, and stores it in the muscles and liver.

Your problem arises when excess carbohydrates are consumed. Once the liver and muscles have stored as much glycogen as possible, the body creates another storage form, FAT. Insulin tells your body not only to store new fat, but also not to release any previously stored fat. **Insulin is the fat storage hormone!**

PROTEIN, on the other hand, stimulates the release of glucagon, which stimulates the liver to RELEASE stored carbohydrates from fat. This encourages your body to use the fat stored around your waist and hips for fuel.

> **IMPORTANT: All carbohydrate breaks down into sugar in our bodies.**

White flour almost immediately turns into sugar. All carbs whether starchy or sweet, quickly turn into glucose in your bloodstream. A bagel can hike your blood sugar as much as a doughnut! Your body has no choice but to release insulin to take care of the sugar.

When you eat too many carbs, insulin levels remain high and you are on a merry-go-round with no getting off! Insulin also works to create new fat cells.
Yes! Fat cells can multiply.

So . . . insulin works to increase the fat we store and decrease the fat we burn.

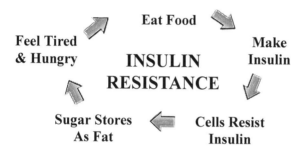

THE ANSWER:
We need to lower our insulin levels and secrete less insulin in the first place!

It is the proverbial Vicious cycle:
When we get fatter, we need more energy and our appetite will increase. We will crave carbs because that is what insulin wants to burn for fuel. The insulin is now in control!

Excess insulin from excess carbs will cause you to gain weight quite quickly. You do not have to eat a lot. This will not happen with protein. The only way to gain weight eating protein is to overeat it. And that is hard to do. Try eating 1000 extra calories of chicken. That is about 5 full chicken breasts!

HOW DID HISTORY GO AWRY?

Studies have long existed that showed that restricting carbohydrates led to significant weight loss. Studies done at University of California, San Francisco, London, England, and Bethesda, MD at the National Institutes of Health all showed that carbohydrates increased hyperinsulinemia and led to obesity.

However, the low-fat diet continued to be touted as the way to lose weight. Instead of saying, watch which fats you eat, doctors and authors said that you should eliminate fat.

Very few people addressed the "elephant in the room" which was that restricting calories and restricting fat DID NOT WORK because people just began to eat more carbs. Dr. Atkins, basically, was correct but because he was not popular among his colleagues, his work was disparaged. He antagonized a group of men who were determined to denounce him. They were not weight loss experts, psychiatrists or even exceptional scientists. They ganged together, prevailed in the court of public opinion, and carbs became popular and fat became the culprit.

Look at what has happened to the American people, including you, since then!

Excess amounts of the hormone INSULIN:
- Makes us accumulate fat
- Tells the liver to convert carbs into fat and releases it into the blood stream as triglycerides
- Causes the kidneys to reabsorb sodium and raises blood pressure
- Causes artery walls to become rigid
- Causes accumulation of HDL into plaque

I repeat, Excess Insulin is making you fat!
It is not difficult to reverse this and lose the weight you want to lose.

YOUR success story starts now!

Chapter 5

Insulin Resistance

The next problem in this losing battle is called
INSULIN RESISTANCE.

The more insulin you secrete, the likelier it is that your cells will become resistant to it. This means that the cells will not "open the door" when insulin comes knocking. Instead, it leaves insulin in your blood stream. Your body senses that there is still insulin in the blood stream and the pancreas releases MORE insulin. More insulin release promotes a greater degree of insulin resistance and we **store more calories as fat.** We are more likely to become insulin resistant as we age. We will store more and more calories as fat. The body continues to pump out more and more insulin, but the cells are still resistant and METABOLIC Syndrome develops. Metabolism is also slowing down.

> So....**even a lean person will get fatter** without increasing calorie intake! The fat accumulates around the waist (where fat cells are most sensitive to insulin). You get the infamous "Belly Fat" or "Muffin Top".

With Insulin Resistance we get fatter, lose control of our blood sugar, develop high blood pressure, HDL cholesterol goes down, and LDL goes up. Metabolic Syndrome, also called Syndrome X, has been associated with Alzheimer's disease and cancer because insulin and high blood sugar can cause brain deterioration. I was at a conference recently where the researchers called Alzheimer's "Diabetes of the Brain".

The brain needs fat (cholesterol) for its building blocks....NOT SUGAR. Also, regarding cancer, excess insulin can cause tumors to both grow and to metastasize. It also leads to many problems in women including infertility, polycystic ovary syndrome (PCOS), fibromyalgia, chronic fatigue, yeast infections and PMS, as well as exacerbating menopausal symptoms.

INSULIN RESISTANCE FACTS:

- Results in weight gain
- The more weight you gain, the greater the insulin resistance
- Can result in high cholesterol and hypertension
- Can lead to a pre-diabetic condition and eventually diabetes
- Is usually coupled with low serotonin levels. You need to limit carbs, but carbs will help with serotonin. This is a Catch-22 which can be circumvented with Supplements

Get the picture? This is as simple as I can put it. Carbs and sweets have to be avoided!

THE FOODS THAT MAKE US FAT MAKE US CRAVE FOODS THAT MAKE US FAT!
Will that help you give them up? It's the only way to stay lean.

THE MECHANISM, AGAIN. . .

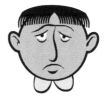

Insulin promotes fat accumulation.

TO GET YOUR BODY TO BURN FAT, DECREASE CARBS & INCREASE PROTEIN

INSULIN IS A BULLY

Do not let him win. Stand your ground! The battle is a worthy one and you will win it!

I made it into a fun game and got so motivated. Giving up sugar for me was relatively easy. Then my husband followed my lead and he lost 37 pounds in just 6 months. AND he was eating more and better than ever!

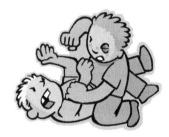

Chapter 6

If I Eat More Protein and Fat, What About My Cholesterol?

Good Question!
Cholesterol is the mother of all the fat molecules in the human body. It maintains brain function, neurotransmitters, nerve endings, regulates mood and helps us digest fat-soluble vitamins. All of our major hormones are made from cholesterol.

**Cholesterol is Essential to the Human Body.
Dietary fat does not cause Weight Gain.**

Cholesterol

It has actually been known since the 1960's that low-fat diets do not significantly lower cholesterol.
A Prime Example: President Eisenhower had a heart attack in 1955. He was put on a low-fat diet eating only oatmeal & skim milk for breakfast. He ate no fat for lunch and low-fat for dinner. His weight and cholesterol went steadily up. His cholesterol rose from 165 in 1955 to 259 in 1961 after FOLLOWING A LOW FAT DIET!
Between 1950 – 1960, some research that supported the conventional wisdom that eating fat caused high cholesterol was given credence.
The researchers believed they were preventing future heart disease, but they did not wait for all the data to be analyzed. Other research was ignored.

The medical community continued to purport that low fat diets were desirable. The myth was born that eating fat raised cholesterol. Therefore, people simply began eating more carbs and sugar.

A Case in Point:
If you replace fat in your diet with carbohydrates...
In other words you have oatmeal and fruit, instead of eggs for breakfast, your LDL cholesterol may go down, but your triglycerides can go up. Also, carbohydrate-rich diets lower HDL (the "good" cholesterol). Low HDL is an excellent predictor for heart attack. You do NOT want a low HDL.

Did you know that LDL and HDL are really not cholesterol?

They are particles that contain the cholesterol and move both it and triglycerides around the blood stream. When insulin is high, LDL particles, which are supposed to be large and benign, become small and dense and attach to the arterial walls to form plaque. A Carbohydrate-rich diet makes LDL small and increases the risk of heart disease...

It also lowers HDL (good cholesterol). When we limit carbs, HDL goes up and LDL particles become larger and more innocuous.

Remember: Large particles of cholesterol are good. Small particles are bad. It is not the cholesterol that is the problem, but the size of the particle.

Studies show that your cholesterol profile IMPROVES when you CUT CARBS.
A recent study published in the Journal of American Medial Association looked at the blood profiles of over 6,100 adults. Those who took in more sugar had low levels of HDL (the good cholesterol) and HIGHER triglycerides. The message was loud and clear: Dietary sugar has a negative effect on cholesterol and triglycerides.

A low carb, protein rich diet should not increase risk of heart disease and will probably PREVENT IT! This is a complete reversal of previous recommendations.

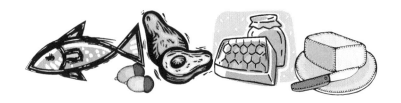

A WORD ABOUT FATS:
Fats are vital to your eating plan
Do NOT be afraid to eat healthy fats ~ It's Biblical!
"Butter and honey shall he eat, that he may know how to refuse the evil and choose the good" Isaiah 7:15

You need fat to <u>regulate mood, energy and hormones</u>. Brain chemical receptors are mainly built from fats! These include:

Omega 3: found in most fish. Flax is also an excellent source. OR purchase fish oil capsules.

Omega 6: found in nuts, seeds, avocados, walnuts, and vegetable oils such as sunflower, safflower. Also found in primrose oil and borage oil as gamma linolenic acid (GLA).

Olive oil is excellent. In fact, consuming olive oil daily has been shown to decrease risk of stroke by about 43%.

NUTS ARE A WONDERFUL SNACK!
Almonds & Walnuts especially
Eating 6 walnut halves are shown to reduce cravings!

> Eating more protein and good fat will not significantly raise cholesterol levels.
> "Numerous studies show that cholesterol from food sources has little effect on levels in your blood".
> Dr. David Katz – O Magazine's Healthy Eating

Chapter 7

Exercise is NOT the Answer

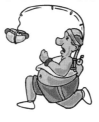

EXERCISE DOES NOT WORK FOR WEIGHT LOSS

Think about it.

We have a proliferation of health clubs in the U.S. and people are just getting FATTER. We have basically seen a "fitness revolution but we are still getting FATTER! IN FACT, USDA guidelines do not suggest that weight can be lost by exercising. Even faithful runners tend to get fatter as the years go by, even those that run more than 40 miles per week. In truth, we do not burn a lot of calories by doing moderate exercise AND it often encourages us to eat more because we think we DID burn those calories. If exercise was truly the answer, construction sites would be full of thin men. And you know that's not true!

Weight gain is not due to sedentary behaviors. Did you ever hear about people who exercise to "work up an appetite?" That's exactly what exercise can do. Your body wants to eat to replenish the energy you just spent.

So…Exercise is good for staying fit, but is not the answer for losing weight. Most people who try to lose weight by exercise are also cutting out unhealthy foods.

Did you ever see a regular jogger or aerobics buff eating a donut after they exercise? No, they are more likely to be drinking some cool water or having something half-way healthy.

That's why these people can stay lean. If they eat the wrong foods, even the distance runner will gain weight.

DO YOU HATE TO EXERCISE?
A recent study released about exercise divided dieters into 2 groups:
Group 1 Dieted only
Group 2 Dieted and exercised 45 minutes 3-5 days/week
The difference was ***only a couple of pounds***!

Diet only group lost 5 – 37 pounds.
Exercise/Diet group lost 8 – 39 pounds.

A compilation of over 43 studies have shown that exercise is not an effective weight loss tool. Of course it is important to your overall health, but walking is just fine.

Forget "EAT LESS, EXERCISE MORE"
WHAT YOU SHOULD REALLY DO IS "EAT BETTER & WALK"

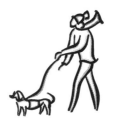

Walking is great because it gets you into a more healthful mood and it won't make you hungrier! A 20 minute daily walk is a great goal.

Quite frankly, the only reason I believe in exercise is to maintain muscle and body tone and for heart health.

I do NOT believe in having to go to the gym to work off bad foods that I have eaten. I am not an extremely active person, but I have maintained my weight for many, many years without a scheduled exercise program.

My main form of exercise is walking, which I do every day. For you, the exercise may help you shrink your fatty areas somewhat faster, but if you EYSS you will not be chained to a gym membership to maintain your desired weight.

Chapter 8

What and How to Eat

a) Always Eat Breakfast

ALWAYS EAT BREAKFAST WITHIN 1 HOUR OF GETTING UP. **Eat a protein food** such as sliced turkey, an egg, cottage cheese, peanut butter, swiss cheese, yogurt or any other protein you choose. Eat a little more than you usually do…more a lunch-like meal. Try this for one week. You will have less bloating and water retention with more protein and your metabolism will increase.

NO SUGAR & NO CEREAL

Those commercials that show people saying "I switched cereals and lost 10 pounds" are silly. You are eating carbs that raise insulin which leads to fat storage.

FAT BUSTER: Eggs are great! They increase metabolism and help burn belly fat. They also contain choline which protects the liver and increases fat loss.

SOME BREAKFAST IDEAS
I actually like eating "lunch" foods for breakfast and I usually eat the same 1 or 2 things every day.
I like:

- Oatmeal mixed with 1-2 tablespoons protein powder. The ONLY way to eat oatmeal, please.
- Dark whole grain toast with peanut butter or almond butter
- Egg whites scramble with some veggies or cheese or some turkey or chicken sausage.
- Protein shake is fine, if that is what you like. Two tablespoons of protein powder provides about 20 grams of protein.
- Sliced turkey with Swiss cheese with a little mustard or mayo rolled into a burrito shape. Yum! 2-3 are filling!
- 2 hard boiled eggs made into an egg salad. Use a little mayo & mustard mix, Thousand Island dressing (my favorite) or your favorite dressing. If you must have it on bread, choose dark whole grain bread.
- Slice of cold pizza (has protein, carbs & fat)
- Greek yogurt (low sugar) w/berries or low sugar jam mixed in. DELISH!

NOTE: We are mostly creatures of habit and that can be a good thing when it comes to eating healthy. Don't feel guilty or lazy. Just pick 1 or 2 breakfasts that you really like and repeat daily. Or eat the same thing every morning.

Now that you have eaten your protein, your brain and metabolism are in a high energy state.

38

 **A note about soy milk:** Soy milk should generally be avoided for three reasons.
#1 It can contain barley malt which is a sugar.
#2 Soy can negatively affect thyroid if ingested too often.
#3 It acts as an estrogen in the body and can contribute to estrogen dominance.

b) What's for lunch?

Lunch or the mid-day meal is the downfall for most of you.

DON'T LEAVE YOUR LUNCHES TO CHANCE.
Figure out 3-5 basic meals and rotate through them. ALWAYS eat lunch and ALWAYS have some protein on hand, even if it is just protein powder that you can mix into something.

NOTE: Don't Avoid Carbs *Entirely*
Complex carbohydrates are essential to helping your brain properly process the tryptophan in protein. Examples are vegetables, legumes or nuts.

FAT BUSTER: Cottage Cheese – Increases L-Tyrosine which helps you feel energetic and full. Has a high casein content which promotes fat loss.

SOME "OK" CARBS (will let you burn fat): Sprouted Grain bread (the darker the better), millett, quinoa, sweet potatoes (even with butter)

GOOD FATS: butter, olive oil, coconut oil, avocados, nuts

NOTE: If there are too many ingredients in a food, **DON'T EAT IT!** It's too processed.

Here are some **SAMPLE LUNCH PLANS FOR YOU** (easy to fix at home or at the office).

LUNCH IDEAS

- Caesar Salad – use only a small amount of the dressing. Make it go further by squeezing extra lemon on the salad.
- OR substitute vinaigrette. Add turkey or chicken
- Chicken breast strips dipped in a little blue cheese dressing
- Egg salad eaten with a fork, no bread
- Tomato and avocado sandwich on Ezekiel bread (see bread note). 1 tablespoon mayo
- Turkey and Swiss cheese on Ezekiel bread
- Tuna sandwich - no extra mayo on Ezekiel bread
- Vegetable omelet
- Greek salad
- Any non-cream soup, unlimited or small portion of creamy style
- Thin crust pizza, 2 slices
- Cobb salad – light ham, extra turkey, light dressing
- Any wrap sandwich, peel off some of the excess wrap. Light dressing
- Turkey roll ups – deli turkey, Swiss cheese, grainy mustard or light layer of mayo.
- Veggie Burger, no bun or just ½ bun
- Side order of meatballs with parmesan cheese
- Cottage cheese mixed with chili powder or other spice OR mixed with seasonal fruit

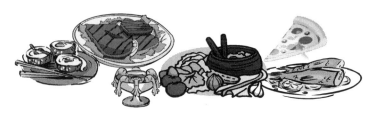

- Yogurt and granola (unsweetened yogurt). My husband loves yogurt, Grape Nuts and fresh blueberries – He mixes a few spoons of flavored yogurt into the unsweetened to make it tastier.
- Shrimp cocktail or shrimp salad
- Crabmeat salad – use low-fat dressing
- Chinese Chicken salad – use half the dressing
- Grilled chicken strips on a green salad or wrapped in a tortilla
- Lettuce wraps – now can be found in frozen section of the market
- Hard boiled eggs
- Low fat potato salad with chicken strips on top
- Any grilled fish with side of potatoes or rice
- Left over steak with some rice or beans
- Tuna on Lettuce with any dressing
- Pita sandwich with chicken, Swiss cheese & tomato
- Small serving of chili with beans and meat
- A baked potato with a topping such as broccoli & cheese
- Triscuits & peanut butter or almond butter
- Baked/ roasted chicken breast w/spinach salad
- Taco salad – Use ½ the dressing. No sour cream
- Chef salad is my favorite
- Any Mexican food minus tortillas and rice. Fajitas are great.
- Sushi Roll

Now that's a lot of choices!

Make your lunches fun! You will soon see that you will stop craving carbs and simply look forward each day to healthy eating. You will find that people may become fascinated with your lunches! Soon you will have disciples!

A NOTE ABOUT BREAD:

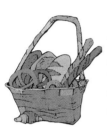

Go "protein style" like they do at "In N Out Burger" put your fillings between lettuce leaves. OR use those very thin wafer type breads that have low carbs like Arnold 100 calorie sandwich thins. I found one called Flatout that is a light flatbread, a kin to a tortilla. It is 100% whole wheat with only 6 carbs per piece and also just 90 calories.
IT'S TASTY TOO!
The only "regular bread I could find that was at all low in carbs was Ezekiel bread, but even that had 11-13 grams of carbs per slice.

FRUIT: Stick to small portions of seasonal fruit.

c) Dinner
Protein PLUS complex carbohydrates.
NO SWEETS.

FAT BUSTERS: Lentils - Contain amino acids that positively affect metabolism of glucose, Spinach – Contains lots of protein, increases muscle tissue and muscle performance. Popeye was right! Increases glucose/carbohydrate metabolism.

FAVORITE DINNER SUGGESTIONS

Baked chicken breasts. Put your spices under the skin and then peel off the skin before serving. (Left-over's are great for breakfast, sliced, with a little mayo, mustard or dressing.)

Pasta sauce with meat. Use spaghetti squash instead of pasta. Bake, boil or microwave it. Scoop out the seeds and shred the strands. Looks just like angel hair pasta and tastes WONDERFUL. Kids love it too! It's magical! Try Marinara sauce with sausage and onion and peppers over spaghetti squash

Salad with grilled chicken, sliced mango & red onion. Squeeze a lemon for the dressing.

Everything But The Kitchen Sink Soup: All your favorite veggies, white beans, spinach, canned tomatoes, lots of spices, prepared low sodium chicken broth. Add sliced chicken or beef cubes or sliced chicken or turkey sausage.

Spicy Stir Fry with brocollini or spinach or both, celery, cherry tomatoes, beef or pork, Chinese garlic sauce (Or use leftover chicken).

Roast a turkey or turkey breast. Serve with fake mashed potatoes made from cauliflower
Grilled or baked vegetables. Throw some sliced chicken on top.
Baked or grilled fish
Vegetarian lasagna
High protein frozen entrée. Amy's Organic or Trader Joe's are good ones.

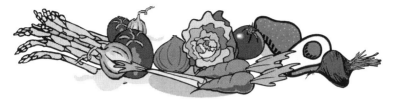

BEST VEGGIES
Broccoli, asparagus, green beans, cauliflower, Brussels sprouts, squash, eggplant, spinach, mushrooms, peppers, tomatoes, turnips, artichoke heart, garlic, cucumbers, celery.
Be careful with corn. It is okay occasionally.

SAUCES & DRESSINGS
Marinara sauce
Emeril's Sauces - usually low in carbs.
I like the dressings that you buy in the produce section that are kept chilled...They contain much less preservative.
Favorites are: Litehouse brand, their "Caesar Caesar" dressing has only 2 carbs and 1 gram of sugar.
Sour Cream is also fine

AN IMPORTANT NOTE ABOUT OVER-EATING
Your stomach is about the size of a 6 ounce can. IF you enlarge it with a huge meal, it takes 3 weeks of small meals to return the stomach to normal size! Yikes . . . now you know what that Thanksgiving dinner can really do! Be careful!

WHAT ABOUT DIET SODAS?
DIET SODA? Is this your "vice"? Do not beat yourself up. I drink them occasionally. They have no carbs. Do not drink more than 3 per day, please.

SNACKS

SNACKS ARE NOT ALL THEY ARE CRACKED UP TO BE! Not everyone needs them.

Perhaps you are not really hungry. We get so used to eating at certain times that it may be a false alarm. Try a little deprivation; it will "reset" your brain. Also, drink water, you may just be thirsty. If you like to snack, time your snacks. Do not indulge in mindless munching.

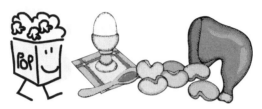

"GOOD" SNACKS

- Deviled eggs made by mixing the yolk with mustard, mayo or Ranch or Thousand Island dressing
- Turkey roll ups
- Shrimp cocktail....can buy some great bargains at wholesale stores
- Sliced baked chicken breast
- Raw almonds or walnuts are wonderful, especially if you have cravings.
- String cheese.
- 10-12 almonds
- Popcorn – 100 calorie bags from the market
- Steamed veggies or raw veggies with ranch dressings or balsamic vinaigrette

PROTEIN BARS THAT I LIKE:

Atkins Chocolate Peanut Butter: 2 net carbs
Atkins Chocolate Coconut: 3 net carbs - these are DELISH!

A BAKED POTATO FOR YOUR EVENING SNACK!
This is a great idea because it will cause your insulin
levels to rise just enough to move tryptophan to your
brain. In the middle of the night your serotonin level will
rise. Sleeping and dreaming are thus wonderfully
enhanced.

In the book, *Potatoes Not Prozac*, the author states that
potatoes can be as effective as an antidepressant in
raising serotonin levels. Also, potatoes have a high
"satiety index" meaning they make you feel satisfied. A
potato has a satiety index of 323 as compared to an
index for ice cream of only 96, pasta of 119 and cookies
120!

**Try my husband's favorite topping—fresh salsa from
the deli section of your market. Butter won't hurt you
if that's your choice. Also, fresh ground
pepper or chili powder is great. I put olive oil &
balsamic vinegar on mine. It's yummy. Be creative!**

**Also, before bed, 1 Tablespoon of peanut or almond
butter (the healthy kind with the oil in the jar). This
really keeps insulin levels steady thru the night.**

**Find your own thin people and ask them
for their best eating tip.
It's a great conversation starter and you
may make a new friend. I love sharing my
tips and others will also.**

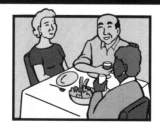

Chapter 9

Cravings Be Gone!

CRAVINGS: If you become hungry AFTER you start thinking about a food, that is the definition of a craving. You feel "driven" to have a cookie, sweet, salty food, late-night snacks, a glass of wine.

It only takes about 15 minutes for a craving to pass. That's not a long time. You can take control!

> "It is easier for an obese person to control his general appetite than to control his cravings for sweets"
> Endocrinologist Hugo Rony

WHY YOU HAVE CRAVINGS:

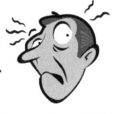

1) Your insulin levels are high and the **insulin wants more sugar.** In other words, the message is "Bring Me Sugar"
2) You are insulin resistant. The glucose is not able to enter your cells and stays in the blood stream instead. Cells are now starved for insulin and send a message to the brain to make more. You crave more sugar because your cells cannot access the insulin that is already in your body.
3) There is an imbalance with your brain chemistry: your serotonin levels are probably low and the brain is looking to raise them with a "pick me up"

People will describe the cravings as actually hearing a "white noise" in their head that actually gets louder and louder until they submit to the craving.

That noise can be silenced FOREVER! Nourishing your brain's neurotransmitters with the correct nutrients and balancing your hormones can completely do the trick! In the meantime, as you Eat Yourself Slender, the cravings will disappear, I promise.

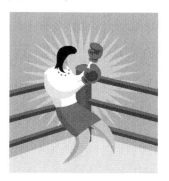

Tips to Give Your Cravings The Cold-Shoulder!

- When a severe craving creeps up on you, eat 6 walnut halves slowly OR eat 1 ounce of a good dark chocolate, savor the taste!
- Eat protein. Grab a slice of turkey or cheese!
- If you crave carbohydrates like pastas and bread, raising dopamine levels can help minimize the cravings. L-Tyrosine is the supplement that raises dopamine.
- Drink lots of water and keep your body hydrated to really help your body brush-off the cravings. Thirst and cravings are related!
- Sleep right! The body resets its hormones during sleep, including insulin and cortisol. Find a way to get an extra hour. Take melatonin to reset your circadian rhythm. Give it time to work, even a month. It is NOT a sleeping pill, but resets the body clock with regular use. For some people it works REALLY fast, but don't give up if it takes longer.

Daily Snack Ideas to Bury Your Cravings!
- Frozen blueberries
- Carrots and hummus dip (or use any crunchy veggie) YUM!
- Popcorn with spice on top. I use chili powder!
- A good brand of dark chocolate (must contain at least 73% cacao to really work)
- A hard boiled egg with some ranch dressing or other condiment will really help.
- WHEN YOU HAVE A CRAVING, EAT SOMETHING THAT IS NOT SWEET.

Try eating a sour pickle or something hot. It can trick your brain into losing the craving. I like to cut up cucumbers, put some olive oil and vinegar and some hot chili peppers on it. By the way, hot foods also raise your metabolism, and that's a GOOD thing!

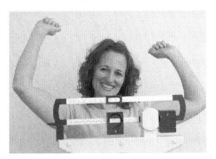

Chapter 10

Supplements to Stop Cravings

Serotonin, Dopamine and GABA (Gamma-Aminobutyric acid) are the neurotransmitters which affect mood and weight gain. If they are not balanced, cravings occur. You, my friend, are probably deficient in one or more of them. There is a self-quiz on page 25 for you to determine your needs.

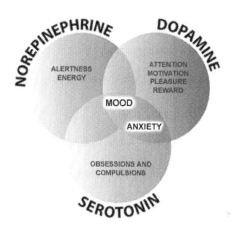

When **SEROTONIN** is normal your mood will be excellent with a sense of well-being. You will be energetic and productive. Your food cravings will be almost non-existent and you will have good control over impulse eating.

When serotonin is low, your ability to control appetite diminishes drastically. This state leads you to overeat, succumb to cravings, and pile on the pounds.

When **DOPAMINE** is normal your metabolism is high. You feel satisfied when you eat and can walk away from the table without overeating. Your cravings for sugar are diminished. You feel focused and in control.

When **GABA** (Gamma-Aminobutyric acid) is normal you feel balanced, not tense, irritable or hungry. You will not succumb to emotional eating. You have control over the impulse to overeat in order to overcome feelings of anxiety or panic.

I have balanced all of these and RARELY ever have cravings.

Chapter 11

SUPPLEMENT SELF-TEST

Let's pinpoint your needs for your weight loss success. Note: You may need more than 1 brain supplement.

IS THIS YOU?

1) I often crave salty foods. I am not hungry in the morning, but I can eat all night long. I look for high carb snacks. I get up at night to snack. I eat small snacks, but lots of them. I have trouble falling asleep at night.

You need SEROTONIN
You are a compulsive eater, over-focused on food / night eater/ carb craver
5-HTP is the supplement for you

2) I need energy. I am consuming excessive amounts of coffee and sugar to get going and keep going during the day.

You need DOPAMINE
You are an impulsive eater with a probable sluggish metabolism
You start each day with good intentions to eat properly, but cannot sustain them
L-Tyrosine is the supplement for you

3) I binge. I over-eat. I have no portion control. I feel addicted to certain foods. When I'm stressed I eat whatever will calm me down. I don't feel like my brain ever tells me to stop eating.

You need GABA
You are an anxious eater. You tend to medicate your feelings of anxiety, tension, nervousness and fear with food.
GABA is the supplement for you

I NEED SEROTONIN:

Low Serotonin Symptoms:
- You will want carbs with every meal
- You crave salty snacks (pickles, olives)
- You crave chocolate or sugary snacks/comfort foods
- Cravings get worse in the late afternoon or evening
- Cravings get worse around time of menstrual cycle
- You get up and eat in the middle of the night
- You have no appetite in the morning
- You overeat at night.
- You eat when stressed
- You consume fewer calories during day, but at night you raid the refrigerator. You are especially looking for high carb snacks
- Panic attacks
- Sad, depressed mood
- You think about food all the time
- You feel deprived
- Compulsive behaviors
- Muscle stiffness, weakness, as in fibromyalgia
- Reduced interest in sex

What Causes Low Serotonin Levels?

- Hormonal imbalance. The decline in hormone levels in women negatively affects serotonin, especially declines in estrogen and progesterone.
- Aging
- Stress – uses up serotonin
- Lack of sleep
- Some prescription drugs can cause permanent damage to the nerve cells that make serotonin
- Lack of sunlight – serotonin levels are lower in the winter as compared to the spring and summer because exposure to light increases serotonin levels
- Not enough fat in the diet
- Insufficient protein in relation to carbs

When Serotonin is High or Sufficient:

- Carbohydrate cravings subside
- Appetite control is restored
- Weight can be controlled
- Mood is elevated
- Sleep patterns return to normal: Research shows that people who suffer an almost uncontrollable urge to binge on carbohydrates late at night are doing it to raise serotonin levels in order to help them sleep
- The ability to cope with cravings for alcohol is strengthened; alcohol abuse can be helped
- Hot flashes can subside (Hence the pharmaceutical surge into creating serotonin-raising drugs for menopause)
- Obsessions and compulsions can be alleviated

- Panic and Anxiety can subside and diminish altogether
- Muscle pain and fibromyalgia may resolve
- Eating disorders can respond positively

SUMMARY
When serotonin levels are normal you will not think about food as much; you will eat smaller portions and feel content, have less cravings, less feelings of hunger. Dieting can lower serotonin levels which creates a vicious cycle.

HOW TO RAISE SEROTONIN LEVELS

SUPPLEMENTS TO ENHANCE SEROTONIN:
5-HTP: (5-hydroxytryptophan) 50-100 mg late in day or at night. Plant-based (from Griffonia simplicifolia seed) 5-HTP is so effective at raising serotonin levels that it has been described as "***the biochemical equivalent of a trip to Hawaii.***" Reduces appetite & cravings.

DHEA: Also helps burn off belly fat (women: 5 – 20 mg   men: 10 – 50 mg)

SAM-e: 400 mg daily. A precursor to serotonin. Excellent to control food craving and for mood. **Works within hours.**

Melatonin: take at night. Suppresses body weight and visceral fat accumulation during the next day (1.2 – 9 mg)

Rhodiola: actually slows the process of serotonin breakdown

Omega 3 Fatty Acids: Assist in raising serotonin levels. Very important for both brain help and hormone production

Vitamin D: elevates mood, causes body to burn fat. Take in a.m. (2000 – 4000 IU)

Zinc: 25-50 mg/day – helps the brain make serotonin from tryptophan. ***Very good for cravings.***

SEROTONIN-ENHANCING HORMONES:
Progesterone: 40 – 80 mg per day
Pregnenolone: 50 mg per day
HGH: available through prescription only

FOODS & SPICES THAT INCREASE SEROTONIN
Avocado
Chicken
Eggs
Turkey
Cottage Cheese
Yogurt
Wheat Germ
Saffron
Nutmeg
Turmeric
Cinnamon
Spearmint
Dill
(These are natural anti-depressants)
Put cinnamon in your tea! – It can reduce cravings for carbs
Eat foods high in tryptophan (the precursor to serotonin)
Use spices in abundance

Also, guess what? Prayer works to increase serotonin levels!

Do drugs like Prozac, Zoloft, Paxil and Lexapro raise serotonin?

These are synthetic drugs which are called **serotonin re-uptake inhibitors (SSRIs).** Here is how they work: They prevent any serotonin in your brain from being re-absorbed by the nerve endings. This keeps whatever serotonin you already have active. **They do not increase your levels** AND THE SIDE EFFECT OF MOST OF THEM IS **WEIGHT GAIN! Why don't the doctors tell us THAT?** Because you would not take them!

I NEED DOPAMINE:

DOPAMINE is a natural amphetamine

When you raise dopamine levels, YOU RAISE YOUR METABOLISM!

For impulsive eaters / sluggish metabolism

An impulsive eater is not thinking of eating, but when they pass food, they will automatically grab it and eat.

Low dopamine symptoms:
- You need more food than a normal person needs to feel "satisfied"
- You often wake up tired
- Your energy spikes after eating, so you constantly snack
- You crave simple carbs (cakes, crackers, chips, pasta, pastries, potatoes, white breads & rice)

LOW DOPAMINE
↓
HIGH CORTISOL
↓
BELLY FAT

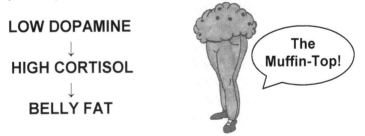

The Muffin-Top!

When Dopamine is low:
- The brain turns to cortisol for energy. When excess cortisol is released, you get puffy and appetite increases. You get bloated and gain weight around the middle because cortisol receptors are located there
- Cortisol increases adrenaline…This makes you feel restless, anxious…not able to sleep at night. Lack of sleep prevents your brain from keeping hormones at correct levels so your hormones are unbalanced and **YOU GAIN WEIGHT**
- Anxiety causes you to crave comfort foods. You might feel "addicted" to certain foods
- Dopamine "kick-starts" your metabolism
- When you have a low metabolism, food automatically accumulates as fat
- Good dopamine levels allow you to experience one helping of a food and then walk away
- Dopamine MAKES YOU FEEL SATISFIED. Your body gets the message that you are full
- Dopamine cuts cravings for sugar
- Your brain is alert & FOCUSED

SUPPLEMENTS TO ENHANCE DOPAMINE:

L-Tyrosine: Raises Dopamine levels and stimulates the body to burn up adipose tissue, promotes satiety (500 – 1000 mg) Dopamine makes you feel satisfied. Your body gets the message that you are full. Dopamine cuts cravings for sugar & caffeine.
Added benefit: Great for the thyroid.
Phosphatidylserine: Increases dopamine and lowers cortisol (200 mg)
Folic Acid: Increases calories burned (400 – 800 mg)
Vitamin D: Helps metabolic syndrome (1000-2000 IU)

CUT OUT SUGAR! SUGAR DEPLETES DOPAMINE

Use Stevia instead of sugar

It has NO calories and is 200-300 times sweeter than sugar. Stevia is a natural dietary supplement which comes from a plant in Brazil.

Keep your Dopamine High

"Get off sugar for your vanity and your sanity!"

FOODS THAT INCREASE DOPAMINE:

Protein increases dopamine.

The amino acids phenlyalanine & tyrosine are found in protein-rich meats, poultry & fish. Beef (get lean cuts), chicken, cottage cheese, eggs, oat flakes, and pork are all good choices.

By the Way: a single serving of cottage cheese (½ cup) greatly increases tyrosine which increases dopamine. Try adding some spices. Personally, I like to add chili powder and turmeric.

OTHER WAYS TO BOOST YOUR METABOLISM:

COFFEE:

- An antioxidant; it facilitates weight loss because it is a diuretic
- Contains soluble dietary fiber, loosens bowels, prevents constipation
- Improves short term memory
- Is not unhealthy. Research shows 2-4 cups per day (small cups) is fine

TEA: Contains L-Theanine which is a relaxant

- Enhances metabolism.
- Helps burn calories & body fat. That is why so many diet products on the market contain green tea.

You can make your own "diet" product. Steep 2 green tea bags and 2 black tea bags. Put the tea in a thermos and sip all day.

I NEED GABA

SYMPTOMS OF GABA DEFICIENCY:
You have a second helping at every meal
You binge at a buffet or you can eat a box of cookies in one sitting
You eat off someone else's plate mindlessly.
You always order dessert just because it is there

GABA is for Calm, Stable Brain Chemistry & Weight Loss
- The brain's calming agent
- Helps maintain proper brain rhythm; keeps brain signals flowing in a calm, steady stream versus shaky "pulses"
- Keeps you feeling balanced (not tense, irritable, hungry)
- Counteracts emotional eating and gives control over feelings that lead to impulsive overeating. No more eating in order to control feelings of panic!
- Stops stressful eating
- Helps with portion control, over-eating
- Cuts cravings for alcohol/drugs/junk food binges
- Can also help migraines, panic attacks, insomnia

GABA is available as a nutritional supplement. With **GABA** you can become one of those people you see eating leisurely and laying down their fork without finishing every morsel on their plate. How wonderful! You are under control!

GABA: 550 mg 1-2 times daily.
I like a product that contains both GABA and L-Theanine 200 mg.   L-Theanine is a mood enhancer & anxiety reducer.

Drink green tea (2-4 cups a day) for calmness, attention & focus.
Decrease caffeine.
Eat complex carbs & high fiber.

OTHER SUPPLEMENTS FOR WEIGHT LOSS IN GENERAL
Natural Progesterone Creme:
Helps balance excess estrogen.
Assists body in using fat for energy
instead of storing it. Use twice daily.

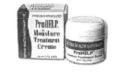

DHEA: Women 5-20 mg Men 10-50 mg Studies show
it reduces abdominal fat, improves mood & depression
, balances blood glucose & enhances fat

Avena Sativa: "Wild Oats" ~ for cravings. The
anecdotal evidence on this product is just amazing.
(Also great for libido)

B Vitamins: B Vitamins aid in the manufacture of
serotonin. Folic acid increases the amount of calories
you burn

WHAT IS MY PERSONAL SUPPLENT REGIMEN FOR WEIGHT CONTROL?

GABA in the morning
L-Tyrosine in the morning
SAM-e in the morning
DHEA in the morning
5-HTP at night
Natural Progesterone crème twice daily
Melatonin at night
Essential Fatty Acids (known as Fish Oils) Buy the best
you can afford and be sure it contains
EPA 720 mg and DHA 480 mg.

To shop for some great supplements at low prices:
www.bhnformulas.com

Chapter 12

How to Sleep Yourself Thin

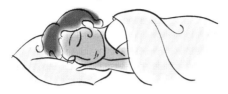

The more tired you are, the heavier you will get.

- Sleep influences the hormones that regulate satiety and hunger…ghrelin & leptin. The levels of both these hormones **fall** when you are sleep deprived.
- Too little sleep translates to hunger, cravings and the feeling of not being fully satisfied.
- **Growth hormone declines with sleep deprivation.** One week of poor sleep inhibits growth hormone. HGH controls the body's proportion of muscle & fat.
- Without proper sleep, you will not have Optimal Serotonin Levels. This leads to food cravings. This leads to more insomnia because you do not make sufficient melatonin. Serotonin is the precursor to melatonin. Melatonin is the sleep hormone which regulates our sleep/wake cycle.
- A sleep-deprived body releases the hormones adrenaline and cortisol and the brains repair and restore cycle does not have enough time to complete its important tasks.
- Proper sleep resets hormones AND helps increase metabolism.
- Sleep lowers cortisol levels. This discourages belly fat accumulation and insulin

THE BOTTOM LINE FOR SLEEP

You need 5 cycles of sleep each night.
Each cycle takes 90 minutes. 5 x 90 minutes = 7 ½ hours.
To determine your bedtime, take the time you need to be up in the morning and count back 7 ½ hours. Then go to sleep at that hour.
You need a 90 min cycle to reach restorative phase: this phase promotes release of neuro-chemicals.

When Dr Oz was asked about his sleeping habits, he said "I set an alarm to go to sleep, not to wake up. I sleep at 10 pm every night and get up just before 6."

SUPPLEMENTS FOR GOOD SLEEP

Progesterone helps because estrogen dominance excites the brain which leads to sleeplessness.
Rub 1/4 tsp of crème on the back or sides of your neck about 1 hour before you go to bed.

Melatonin: 1.2 mg—6 mg 45 minutes-1 hour before bedtime
Choose a consistent bedtime to reset your internal body clock.

I really like transdermal or sublingual melatonin as it works best for most people vs. the pill form.

NOTES:

Chapter 13

Hormone Balance is Key in Weight Loss

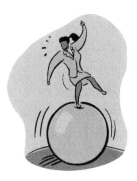

Yes, yes, yes. This is so true!

As we have discussed, high insulin (a hormone) is bad. The other hormone that controls fat distribution is estrogen (in both men and women). We need to get both of these hormones balanced. <u>All hormones communicate with each other.</u> Hormones and fat cells are connected by a network within the body that <u>synchronizes appetite, metabolism, digestion and elimination & detoxification.</u>

When hormones become unbalanced, the entire system becomes unbalanced and can cause weight gain and food cravings along with your other menopausal symptoms such as hot flashes.

WHAT DO HORMONES HAVE TO DO WITH WEIGHT GAIN?

- Hormones affect appetite
- Hormones affect metabolism
- Hormones affect fat storage
- Hormonal imbalance can lead to depression, food binges & uncontrollable cravings
- Hormonal imbalance, particularly low progesterone, can lead to thyroid disorders. Progesterone and Thyroid are "best friends!" Low thyroid leads to weight gain
- Birth control pills can cause weight gain because they contain high levels of hormones

Note: **You may do just fine by using natural progesterone crème to restore hormonal balance.**

Many women have lost a dress size or more after just months of using natural progesterone to balance estrogen dominance. Others, may have a serotonin, GABA or dopamine deficiency which is blocking efforts to lose weight.

HIGH INSULIN LEVELS in women lead to increased testosterone levels. This blunts estrogen effects which can lead to no ovulation and decreased progesterone production.

PROGESTERONE DEFICIENCY can trigger sugar cravings because GABA is low. INSULIN RESISTANCE CAUSES A DROP OF SEROTONIN LEVELS. You eat sugar to feel good, but this increases Insulin Resistance which leads to more cravings and eventually addiction to sugar.

Also **increased insulin** leads to increased adrenaline and cortisol levels, which means that you now have three hormone levels that are elevated beyond their normal ranges.

DID YOU KNOW?
There are 35 Symptoms of Hormone Imbalance:
1. Hot flashes, flushes, night sweats and/or cold flashes, clammy feeling
2. Irregular heart beat
3. Irritability
4. Mood swings, sudden tears
5. Trouble sleeping through the night
6. Irregular periods; shorter, lighter periods; heavier periods, flooding; shorter cycles, longer cycles
7. Loss of libido
8. Vaginal dryness
9. Crashing fatigue
10. Anxiety, feeling ill at ease
11. Feelings of dread, apprehension, doom
12. Difficulty concentrating, disorientation, mental confusion
13. Disturbing memory lapses
14. Incontinence, especially upon sneezing, laughing
15. Itchy, crawly skin
16. Aching, sore joints, muscles and tendons
17. Increased tension in muscles
18. Breast tenderness
19. Headache change: increase or decrease
20. Gastrointestinal distress, indigestion, flatulence, gas pain, nausea
21. Sudden bouts of bloat
22. Depression (see note)
23. Exacerbation of existing conditions
24. Increase in allergies

25. Weight gain (see note)
26. Hair loss or thinning, head, pubic, or whole body; increase in facial hair
27. Dizziness, light-headedness, episodes of loss of balance / disorientation
28. Changes in body odor
29. Electric shock sensation under the skin and in the head
30. Tingling in the extremities
31. Gum problems, increased bleeding of gums
32. Burning tongue, burning roof of mouth, bad taste in mouth, change in breath odor
33. Osteoporosis (after several years)
34. Changed in fingernails: softer, crack or break easier
35. Tinnitus: ringing in ears, bells, 'whooshing,' buzz, etc.

Wow!
That's a lot of correctible symptoms

HORMONE FACTS FOR YOU:

- Perimenopausal and Menopausal weight gain is an increasing problem due to environmental estrogens.
- Weight is gained in the mid-section, causing a change in body shape. The stomach area becomes rounder and it is difficult to re-distribute the weight.
- About 90% of women gain weight between the ages of 35 and 55. This can be 40 pounds or more! I have seen 100 pound weight gains!
- Research shows that fluctuations in your hormones and ingestion of carbohydrates, not over-eating, are usually the culprit.
- Women who have had a hysterectomy (called surgical menopause) can experience a more rapid and extreme weight gain.
- This weight gain has been termed the "middle-aged spread" and women have been told to just accept it.
- Men who are exposed to xeno-estrogens and/or eat too many carbs can experience drastic weight gain that will not budge.

So, men and women need to get hormones balanced so that they do not have estrogen dominance. Many of you are already using a natural progesterone crème. **If you need further help in this area you can request the free booklet, *Natural Progesterone For You* or call us at 877-880-0170 we want to help you.**

Tips From Your *Thin* Friends

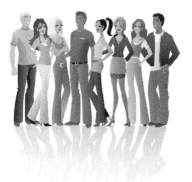

- Spice It Up! Go to a healthy market like Trader Joe's, Henry's or Whole Foods. Get some great new spices, rubs, salsas, hot sauces, even light gravies. Also, get some really good mustard. YUM! Spices help burn calories & raise metabolism
- Only eat bread in a sandwich. No toast! Toast is now "toast" in your kitchen
- For salad dressing, get some good balsamic vinegar & good quality olive oil. Make a dressing using the vinegar, olive oil, mustard and a little Stevia if you like a sweeter dressings. I go to the store and buy a really good fresh dressing – the kind you find in a jar in the produce section. Then I dilute it with balsamic vinegar or lemon and kick it up with some spices. I make a couple of tablespoons at a time. ½ the calories and so DELISH!

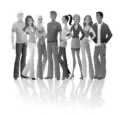

- Just plain old hungry? My Number One go-to food is pizza. Yes, that's right! Ask for whole-wheat, thin crust, light cheese (I like extra sauce) and pile on the veggies. (The veggies actually help fight wrinkles and the tomatoes in the sauce fight sun damage for your skin). Also, this is a good protein low-fat snack without a lot of calories. One piece is about 200 calories and you will feel FULL!
- No baggy clothes! Wear your thinnest clothes so you can feel that waistband. Studies show loose clothing inhibits weight loss
- Eat early in the day, something within first 30 – 45 minutes of rising
- Increase fiber intake. This helps the body excrete excess estrogens
- Avoid artificial sweeteners
- Don't over-exercise. This depletes serotonin and stresses metabolism. The stress hormone increases and affects other hormones. If you feel hungry after exercising, you have actually "over-exercised"
- Eat good fats daily. Low-fat eating prompts your body to hang on to any extra body fat. Good fats also help balance hormones
- 1 Tbs. Flaxseed oil per day is a wonderful source of linolenic acid which promotes hormone balance.

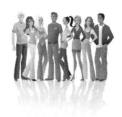

- Walking & stretching can help raise serotonin levels and improve well-being
- Avoid alcohol when starting your plan. It is a brain depressant and can perpetrate cravings. Wait until you feel balanced before you consume any alcoholic beverages
- Avoid anti-depressants: They treat the symptoms not the cause. One of the main side effects is WEIGHT GAIN!
- **LET THERE BE LIGHT**! Increase melatonin production by keeping your circadian rhythm in sync. Get 20 minutes of bright light daily. Try drinking you're A.M. coffee or tea outside. People tend to lose weight in the summer because the increased light boosts their serotonin so carbohydrate cravings naturally decrease
- Turn off most lights ½ hour before bedtime. Do not turn on lights if you get up in the middle of the night. Light interrupts melatonin production & you start from ground zero with your melatonin
- Looking at healthy foods promotes cravings for healthy foods. Consider putting photographs, pictures, or calendars depicting healthy foods in your home or office. It works for me and my staff!
- Drink water with lemon when eating out instead of ordering a restaurant beverage

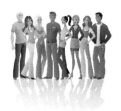

- If you experience cravings, eat 6 walnut halves OR 1/2 oz chocolate (not both!) These trigger your brain "I am no longer hungry" via the vagus nerve. It really works!
- Eat hummus as a dip on fresh vegetables. There are some great varieties available. I like Spicy Hummus! Or, add hot sauce to plain hummus
- Eat lots of spinach! Loaded with protein
- Eat tiny grape tomatoes as a snack Yum! Dip in ranch dressing or hummus
- Eat apples with almond butter. Almond butter at night helps keep blood sugar levels stable.
- Sniff peppermint every 2 hours. A recent study showed that people who did this were not as hungry as non-sniffers and, even better, they ate 2,800 fewer calories per week! That's enough to lose close to a pound
- Eating slower means fewer calories - Make dining an experience…not a race
- Make your Restaurant meal two meals in one. Divide it the minute it comes to the table and ask for a box
- Do not do anything except eat when you sit down for a meal. Do not read, watch TV, talk on the phone, work, etc. Be aware of the food you are eating
- Do not keep food in any other room besides the kitchen

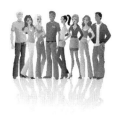

- If you are in the habit of going right to the kitchen when you go home, map out an alternative "route" in your house
- Gum works as an appetite suppressant and also appears to curb cravings for sweets
- Always eat with a fork and spoon. This helps with food selection. You cannot eat salad or chunky soup with your hands and those are healthy choices
- Cut down on the dressing on salads. I took a bite of my friend's salad and could not believe how much dressing she had on it! Gloppy and over-powering! Don't let this be you
- Start small... one change at a time is a great strategy. Maybe just cutting back on the cream and sugar in your coffee
- Limit anything fried to once per week
- Replace ground beef with ground turkey
- If you do not really love it, do not eat it!
- Never eat out of a bag or box. Take out a measured or counted quantity of food and put it in a bowl
  A no-brainer!
- Give left-over party food to guests to take home
- Never skip a meal to conserve calories
- Bake yams in their skins. Mash and season with roasted garlic and herbs
- Floss your teeth like crazy instead of eating

Chapter 14

GET MORE WILLPOWER!

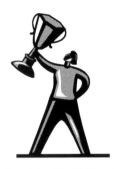

Blood Glucose is linked to Self-Control

A new study suggests that blood glucose is an important part of self-control and willpower. **Keeping glucose regulated improves self-control.** Self-control is the capacity to override one's impulses and automatic or habitual responses. Researchers have been finding that self-control steadily declines during the day because glucose problems increase as the day progresses and willpower vanishes. **Researchers found that when glucose levels remained high all day, willpower suffered.**
Coping with stress requires self-control, and after coping with everyday stresses, people are less successful at self-control.

THE SECRET TO MORE CONTROL:
Keep your glucose normal, available and non-fluctuating. This leads to improved self-control, better focus and the ability to cope with stress. A glycemic index chart of foods can help you. Also, I love a product called PGX crystals which regulates insulin levels during the day. A product called Chromate is also great.

You must eat properly to keep glucose stable. Also, we must be willing to feel hungry sometimes in lieu of eating high sugar offerings. When I was growing up and it was just before the mealtime, I would sometimes complain to my mother "I'm hungry", looking for a snack. She would simply reply "Good, we'll be eating in an hour" Smart lady!

Also, I like to refer to that hungry feeling as my Lean Machine feeling....let's get some work done here....I'm feeling powerful. And I am. I have power over my hunger.
In essence, that is WILLPOWER!

> **"I can do all things through Christ who strengthens me." Philippians 4:13**
>
> **"He gives power to the weak, and those who have no might He increases strength."**
> **Isaiah 40:29**

Chapter 15

What's In Your Kitchen?
HOW TO BEAT THE
SUGAR MONSTER

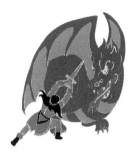

Let's Take a Look and see where sugar is lurking in your house!

FATS
- Bottled salad dressings
- Imitation mayonnaise or sour cream
- Margarine
- Non-dairy creamers
- Pressurized whipped cream
- Cream substitutes, flavored and unflavored

HIGH SUGAR FOODS
(Some you will recognize, some will surprise you!)
- Flavored popcorn
- Cocoa
- Fruit butters
- Fruit leathers
- Jello - this is pure sugar!
- Granola bars or granola
- Energy bars - some are just "dressed up" candy! Also, many contain chemicals

- Honey
- Ice cream
- Jams, jellies, marmalade (except low-sugar versions)
- Molasses
- Processed yogurt, flavored yogurt. choose Greek Yogurt
- Sherbet
- Syrups
- Fruit juice: 12 ounces of most have the same amount of sugar as a 12 oz soda
- Gatorade (14 grams of sugar in 8 ounces)
- Ensure
- Soy milk, rice milk. Almond milk is best choice but still has sugar.
- Carnation Instant Breakfast- 22 grams per serving!
- Bacon
- Muffins
- Flavored vinegars (not balsamic, but flavored)
- Tonic water - LOTS of sugar in it!
- Syrup sweetened fruit
- Anything "fat free"
- Croissants, toast, bagels
- BBQ sauce
- Hoison sauce / oyster sauce
- Ketchup
- Relishes
- Sweet pickles
- Gravies

Banish these hidden sugar foods and you will see a steady weight loss, feel more energy, have a better mood and better sleep. I PROMISE!

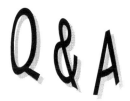

Q: I am a widow. I'm lonely and I do not like to cook for myself. What can I do?
A: This is *exactly* what you should be doing for yourself! You don't have to cook "serious" dishes. Just have healthy food on hand. You can be one of those 90 year old ladies who are slender, full of energy, and a great example to the "young uns". Eat the same healthy foods over & over. It won't seem so over-whelming.

Q: Should I count carbs?
A: Do you want to count carbs? If you do, fine. Keep your net carb intake low. Stay below 10 grams for any given item. When you read labels, you can **subtract** fiber and sugar alcohol because these will not cause insulin spiking.
The result is the net carbs in the product.
Two examples: on my bag of Pitted Plums I have, 1 servings = 11 grams of sugar.
Fiber = 3 grams. That is a NET of 8 grams.

Atkins Chocolate Peanut Butter Bar Total carbs 22 grams Fiber 10 grams Sugar Alcohols 10 grams. Subtract the fiber and sugar alcohol and the NET is just 2 grams.

Q: What about Sugar Substitutes?
A: Sweeten foods with Stevia. Stevia rebaudiana bertoni is the leaf from a shrub in the chrysanthemum family that is grown in South America and Asia. Stevia is about 150 to 300 times sweeter than sugar, has zero calories, and doesn't raise blood sugar levels.

However, if you reach a plateau, cut out all sugar substitutes.

Q: "I have not lost weight in a week"
A: Scale didn't budge? Take measurements.
Protein increases lean muscle mass. This increase can keep you at the same weight, so you think you are on a plateau. This is NORMAL. Don't panic. The scale can lie but measurements won't.
  Best places to measure:
- Thigh
- Waist
- Hips

Q: Can you recommend any other low carb diet books?
A: Yes! Here you go:
Dr. Atkins Diet Revolution
The Scarsdale Medical Diet
The Zone
Protein Power
Sugar Busters
The South Beach Diet

Q: Should I use the glycemic index?
A: Some of you have asked me about this and it does have popularity among some medical doctors and authors of diet books. It actually comes down to common sense when choosing your foods, but here is how the GI works.

The GI is a numerical system of measuring how quickly a food triggers a <u>rise</u> in blood glucose. The score of pure glucose = 100. All other foods are measured in relation to this.

In other words, WHAT IS THE SUGAR CONTENT OF THIS FOOD? The Glycemic Index will tell you.

The higher the GI number, the more the glucose is released in a surge which triggers dramatic spikes in blood sugar. The lower the GI, the more gradual the release of the glucose. LOWER GI IS BETTER! If you want to use the GI index as a tool, stay away from foods with a GI of 70 or higher because they provide the heftiest surge in blood sugar. Choose foods with a GI of 55 or less because they trigger a small, steady rise in blood sugar. These are most vegetables, legumes, whole grains, and low-sugar foods. You can judiciously select foods with a GI between 56-69, which cause a slightly higher glycemic response. These can be your TREATS. Reduce White flour foods as best you can. If you simply must eat a "white" food, choose those that give you the <u>least</u> pleasure so no addiction is triggered.

SUGGESTION:
For the first 3 weeks, avoid high glycemic fruits and veggies: corn, cantaloupe, raisins, bananas, papayas, grapes, watermelon, potatoes, beets, mango. Then you can introduce them in small portions.

Q: What can I use in place of bread and pasta? I love to grab toast or a bagel in the morning and a sandwich at lunch and I like pasta or rice at dinner.
A: This is too many carbs and your body will have no choice but to store fat. Re-train your Brain! Quinoa tastes like pasta. Spaghetti squash looks like pasta and you can eat copious amounts of it. Vegetable lasagna is excellent.

Soon you will not miss pasta as a regular food. It will be your treat. I was actually a pasta-holic, eating it daily. I am very content with my new choices.

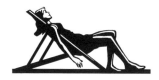

Q: "I cannot follow a diet. I have adrenal fatigue"
A: You need to get off sugar and eat more protein! Don't use sugar to bolster your energy. This will backfire because you are driving tired adrenals even harder. Then your cortisol levels become exhausted and your immune system lies down on the job. Sugar cravings increase.

Chronic fatigue & fibromyalgia can occur when adrenals lose the ability to self-regulate. Cortisol levels are low during the day and high at night. Insomnia occurs. Chronic pain can occur. Auto-immune diseases can occur and your thyroid can suffer.
This plan is excellent for you!

Q: My husband eats too fast, isn't this bad for you?
A: Yes, actually. Eat slowly and ENJOY your food. Try to chew each bite 20 times. 30 times is even better. Try it . . . its fun and relaxing. It's a good example to your family. Do you have family members who lower their heads and don't come up for air until they are done? They will eat too much and be headed for a lifetime of weight issues. Stop it now! Set a timer to get used to eating slowly. Don't go for second helpings until you have waited 15 minutes. You may find you are really full and do not need more.

Q: Why can't I buy serotonin pills to stop my cravings?
A: Serotonin is not sold as a supplement because it cannot easily cross the blood brain barrier.
5-HTP is a natural serotonin precursor and easily crosses from the blood stream into the brain. See the chart below:

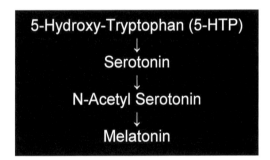

5-Hydroxy-Tryptophan (5-HTP)
↓
Serotonin
↓
N-Acetyl Serotonin
↓
Melatonin

As you can see, once serotonin is made, the pineal gland is able to convert it at night into melatonin, the sleep-inducing hormone so better sleep occurs also.

Q: Is there a blood test for serotonin levels?
A: The blood test for serotonin is complex and not routinely available in Doctors offices. Since serotonin levels in the blood fluctuate throughout the day, the test would not be practical. Serotonin can also be checked by spinal fluid via a spinal tap: a very invasive procedure. Instead, go by your symptoms!

Q: Is there a test for insulin resistance?
A: Yes, but it is complicated and expensive. A recent study has confirmed that when a woman's waist is bigger than 35 inches, she most probably has Insulin Resistance. For a man it is 40 inches. Women with polycystic ovarian syndrome (PCOS) usually are insulin resistant. If you gave birth to a baby 9 pounds or more or you weighed 9 pounds or more at birth, you may be resistant. African-Americans have triple the risk.

Q: Can I take 5-HTP if I am taking another anti-depressant drug?
A: I have seen some great articles that suggest that these products can help alongside anti-depressants and even help people wean off them. However, you must check with your doctor or qualified medical professional since clinical depression is a serious disorder. You should NEVER abruptly stop any anti-depressant medication. It appears that you can add SAM-e if you are taking an anti-depressant.

Q: What if I am on a diet that is not working well for me?
A: Is it low calorie? Researchers from the University of Oxford found that in just
3 weeks on a **low calorie diet,** people's tryptophan levels dropped significantly. In other words, **dieting leaves you vulnerable to low serotonin levels which affect mood.** Therefore, you run the risk of depression or future binge eating. A good solution is to take a planned break from your current diet once a week. This can be in the form of a "free meal" or a day to just indulge in a few healthy high calorie choices.

Q: What can I eat if I am hungry late at night?
A: You are going to break the cycle of unhealthy late-night snacking.

It is best to go to bed without a heavy snack. Try eating dinner a little later or eat more for your dinner.

Here are some good choices:
Baked Potato
Peanut or almond butter
A product containing chocolate called Sleep Squares (also contain melatonin)
Some sliced roasted turkey
Sliced peppers or carrots with hummus
Herb tea is a good choice. Mighty Leaf makes one called Chocolate Mint Truffle that is great
Sugar Free hot chocolate
One lady told me she whitens her teeth at night when she feels a snack attack coming on.

Q: I eat when I am stressed. Help!

A: The higher your cortisol levels, the more you will crave carbs. Don't give in. Choose protein instead. Or eat some Greek Yogurt with a little sugarless jam mixed in.

Rhodiola Rosea is a great adaptogenic herb that reduces daily stress and also enhances mental performance as it helps with weight reduction. Take 1 capsule daily. Look for a 500 mg capsule.

Q: My husband loves carbs and this will be so difficult with all of his chips and bread around the house and his expectation of carbs with dinner.

A: Try to enlist him as part of your team. Ask him to support you in your sugar challenge. When men give up sugar, carb cravings often quickly disappear. For some reason, this is easier for men than it is for women.

If he won't cooperate, portion control! Make only enough carbs for him.

OR, for a couple of weeks get some yummy frozen dinners. If he has pasta, you have chicken. There are some really nice frozen entrees available now...just watch for high sodium content. You want to avoid that.

Q: What can I do about celebrations I am invited to....birthdays, holidays?

A: Go for It! The next day, just do an all-protein day. Now, that does not mean you should pick and nibble all day. If it is Thanksgiving, just indulge in your favorite meal items like turkey, stuffing and pie. No chips or dips. You will be fine!

Q: What can I eat on vacations?
A: Vacations are going to be a great time for you because you are finally EATING and not trying to count calories and take all the fun out of the experience. For breakfast, no carbs, but you can have egg white omelets, Canadian bacon, poached eggs, fruit, cheese, yogurt and all good condiments including sour cream. There are some phenomenal omelets you can make or order out. The rest of the day, carbs are okay and fat is fine. Remember, the only bread you can have is in a sandwich. I like to order jumbo sandwiches and ask the waiter to put the ingredients on a bed of lettuce and give me a nice dressing. I get jealous looks from other tables, as in "Why didn't I think of that?" One tip...stay out of the minibar...no good will come of it! Finally, have your home fridge or freezer stocked with protein-rich food for when you come home. I always freeze a bunch of meatballs for myself.

The day after returning from a trip or vacation is an all-protein day. Choose high protein, no dairy or alcohol. All snacks must be protein. It works! If you have gained some weight in 6 days, you can lose it in one day. Going back to work? Bring your protein with you. If you order lunch, choose a Chicken Caesar salad . . . no croutons, after all they are just stale bread! Use a nice balsamic vinaigrette or mix it with the Caesar dressing. You are back on track . . . No harm done!

Q: What about eating in airports?
A: This is not as difficult as you may think. Go for a slice of pizza (add lots of hot crushed pepper...turns up the metabolism). Starbucks has a chicken sandwich that is good. Just eat 1/2 the bread, or split it with someone. Or get some dressing and eat it with a knife and fork. California Pizza Kitchen is in a lot of airports and they have great salads. Any grilled chicken or chicken Caesar salad will be an excellent choice.

Q: What are your tips for eating out in restaurants?
A: Enjoy yourself, but NO Bread basket! I'd rather see you have a bread fight with your fellow diners than eat that bread! Ask for bread sticks and dip those in the butter or olive oil. Give up the bread, but reward yourself with a nice baked potato with yummy olive oil or butter. Or hold the starch altogether and get double veggies. My husband has been doing this for a year and the chefs have made him some fabulous veggies because he asks so nicely. Sometimes I just get 2 appetizers or a beefed up salad....in other words, choose a salad and ask for extra chicken or some fish on top.

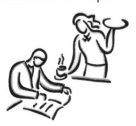

Eat slowly and chances are you will not want dessert. Avoid those price-fixed meal offerings where dessert is included.
If you must have some, choose the lowest sugar chocolate offering available. Get some peppermint tea or other specialty tea and sip it with gusto!

In *Asian* restaurants, get steamed dishes with sauce on the side. Moo shoo chicken is good. Brown rice, only. No sweet and sour dishes. Order soup, light on the noodles, extra veggies. Easily done by the kitchen staff. Hot and sour soup is also good. Drink lots of water during or after, as this food tends to be higher in sodium. *Greek* food is great. Order Greek Salad, grilled kabobs. Ask them to only give you half the rice and some extra salad or veggies.

Italian: Get a salad or minestrone soup. I order a double order of meatballs and a side of angel hair pasta with marinara. Another great choice is a vegetarian pizza or meatball pizza.

Mexican: Skip the chips, ask for some sliced jicima and dip that in the salsa OR just take a handful of chips and send the basket away. Order entrees without the burrito or tostada shell. Get all beans, vegetables and protein. Use sour cream and avocado and enjoy. This is a really healthy outing for you.

Q: How much water should I drink?
A: Water helps weight loss. It appears to have a stimulating effect on metabolism. Also, the more water you drink, the less bloat you will have. Ask a slice of lemon or lime. I mix unsweetened cranberry juice in water. So pretty with the lemon in it! Try for 6 glasses per day if you can.

Q: What about alcohol?
A: Many people do not want to give up their glass of wine or their cocktail. Just remember, alcohol metabolizes as a carb. Limit yourself to 1 drink per day, 2 at the most.

Chapter 17

Take the Sugar Challenge

Before you begin your Sugar Challenge; Some Steps to Take

- Try finding a buddy
- Tell your friends and relatives what you are doing and ask them NOT to tempt you with sweets
- Get your children to help you police the foods at the super market. This is how I turned my son into a proverbial Sugar Cop! If I tried to sneak a sugary substance into my grocery cart, he would take it out.
- Ask a family member join the program with you
- Remind yourself that you are making a WONDERFUL, POSITIVE change in your life. You are Detoxing from a DRUG and you will feel great!
- Remember that you are in control! NOT the sugar!
- If you like to write, keep a journal. Your story can be valuable to help someone else someday. You could even self-publish it!

 FIRST STEP: 2 weeks off!

Here are the rules for the 2 week challenge. Do as many of them as you can! There is no failing! Any elimination of sugar is a good thing. But try to make me proud of you! ☺

Attempt to eat little or no sugar for 6 days, then give yourself a "Reward Day" on the weekend. After 6 days off sugar, you will begin to notice how SWEET sugar really is!

Do not worry about calories during this 14 days. You are ONLY going to watch your sugar and BREAK THE SUGAR ADDICTION!

TELL SOMEONE WHAT YOU ARE DOING!
ASK SOMEONE TO BE YOUR

"SUGAR SHERIFF"

1. Read all labels. Do not eat any food or serving of food that has over 9 grams of sugar. Become a food detective. To reduce sugar, you have to know where it is lurking!
2. Stop adding sugar to your tea or coffee. Try this for 2 weeks! If you simply cannot, at least cut the amount IN HALF! No artificial sweeteners. They increase cravings
3. Drink sugar-free herbal teas
4. Eliminate white rice, white bread, white pasta. They all convert to sugar in the body
5. Do not buy "Fat-free" foods. (Usually loaded with sugar)
6. Cut down on salt. Salty foods lead to cravings for sweets
7. Substitute Raisin Bread for breakfast if you are used to a Danish, scone or muffin
8. Still need toast? Melt some cheese and put it on top of your toast. You can melt it right in the microwave in a few seconds. This gives you protein

ISN'T THIS FUN? LET'S KEEP GOING!

9. Reward yourself with chocolate at the end of the day. Make sure it is at least 73% cacao otherwise it is too sugary
10. Keep nuts, cheese, popcorn, whole grain crackers around for snacks. Be careful of trail mix which can contain sugary components
11. No bakery goods – even low fat. I gave up bran muffins which you would think were healthy, but now if I even sample one I can tell how sugary they are!
12. Try an unsweetened nut butter from the store. Check the sugar grams in peanut butters and be careful!
13. Give up ham and bacon for breakfast. They contain sugar!
14. Eat sliced peaches, strawberries, blueberries as your treat. They may seem expensive, but eat them slowly and savor them. You deserve it!
15. Watch your milk intake! Milk contains sugar. Read the label! Rice milk and soy milk are sugary also
16. Stay away from fruit juice. Even the "Unsweetened" ones contain lots of sugar. I know, this surprised me too
17. No commercial salad dressings for these 2 weeks.! I bring my own to the restaurant in a little glass bottle. If you have some in your fridge, thin them out with some oil or vinegar
18. Salsa makes a good dressing
19. Choose a nice ripe avocado for a snack when you have a craving
20. Ketchup is LOADED with sugar. Thin it out with some salsa or some sour crème or your own creative choice
21. Eat pizza for a snack! Has both fat & protein to satisfy you

22. Eat carrots & hummus. There are some wonderful flavors of hummus. You are crunching & dipping and you will NOT hurt yourself sugar-wise or calorie wise
23. Do not eat dry-roasted nuts, they contain sugar
24. No soft drinks! Choose iced-tea!
25. Be careful with alcohol. It acts like a pure sugar in the body. Dilute it!
26. No syrup sweetened fruit. If you have some, strain it and rinse
27. No bagels! The flour converts to sugar in the body and will be stored as triglycerides otherwise known as fat
28. Find some good canned soups that are hearty and rich. Check label for sugar
29. Eat turkey and Swiss cheese rolled up with some mustard as a snack. There are countless varieties of mustard and they do not contain sugar!
30. Watch out for protein bars. Many are loaded with sugar. Look for the Atkins brand
31. Increase protein. Are you getting the message loud and clear? It is important.
32. Microwave a baked potato for a snack. Top with Sour Crème, salsa, butter, guacamole or olive oil. This is a great bedtime snack because it helps raise serotonin levels
33. If you are cravings sweets, cook a yam or sweet potato
34. Do not overdo it with fruit for these two weeks. Maybe two pieces per day

Sweeteners; *The Good, The Bad, The Ugly*

Sugar in its Many Forms:
Yup! These can all be bad!

Agave syrup or nectar
Barley malt
Brown Sugar
Glucose
Granulated sugar
Cane syrup
High Fructose Corn Syrup
Confectioners sugar
Table sugar
Lactose
Liquid cane sugar
Sucrose
Dextrose Chicory Syrup
Tapioca syrup
Splenda

Fructose
Maple Syrup
Powdered sugar
Cane sugar
Raw sugar
Rice syrup
Honey
Sugarcane syrup
Date sugar
Turbinado sugar
Unrefined sugar
Corn Syrup
Maltose
Blonde Sugar

That's right, no Splenda. Splenda is found in over 4,000 foods & beverages on the market. What is it? Splenda is a chemical! Yes, chlorine is forced into an unnatural bond with a sugar molecule substituting sucrose atoms with chlorine atoms. Splenda begins as a sugar and ends up as a synthetic chemical! Also, it can act as an estrogen mimic in the body. Watch for it and AVOID it!

Aspartame (Equal, NutraSweet) can deplete chromium and lead to insulin resistance. It can also increase sugar cravings because it blocks production of serotonin. Sweet'n Low is saccharin, a petroleum derivative. Other names are Necta Sweet and Sweet Twin

What about honey? Honey is a natural sweetener but has more calories and is actually sweeter than sugar, it also raises the blood sugar even more that white sugar. It does have some medicinal benefits and contains small amounts of minerals.

Agave syrup or nectar is made from the fruit of the agave, a cactus-like plant native to Mexico. It is roughly 75 percent sweeter than sugar.

BEST SOURCES OF SWEETENER:
Date "sugar" is made from pulverized dried dates. It is not refined like sugar. It also contains fiber and is high in many minerals. Because the "sugar" is just dried fruit, it is allowed on sugar-restricted diets.
Blackstrap Molasses is 65% sucrose but does have minerals including iron and calcium so is more nutritious than sugar.
Stevia has thirty times the sweetness of sugar but it does not raise blood sugar like other caloric sweeteners.
Sweet Perfection: This is a new sweetener that can be used like sugar in tea, coffee, and baking. It is chicory root ground to a powder that is very high in soluble fiber and looks and tastes exactly like sugar. It will not cause insulin surges.

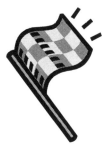

<u>ARE YOU READY TO TAKE THE SUGAR CHALLENGE? LET'S GO!</u>

1. BE EXCITED FOR YOURSELF! You are embarking on a new adventure. You are taking your body on VACATION! Sugar is an unhealthy, destructive, addictive habit that will rob years from your life.

2. Make yourself a slogan. Mine was "I don't eat sugar" I actually was in one of those large warehouse type stores where they give samples. A woman was literally chasing me with a sample of peanut M&Ms on a tray. I simply said "I don't eat sugar" and it REALLY helped me not to even try one. Yours could simply be "I'm cutting down on my sugar". Whatever sounds reasonable to you.

3. Congratulate yourself at the end of each day. Ask someone else to congratulate you, too.

4. Pick a Bible verse or inspirational verse that makes you feel good (and STRONG!)

5. Remind yourself. I am going to be less fat, have more energy and have new brain power!

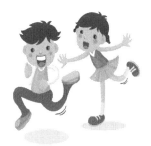

Chapter 18

How to Keep or Get Your Kids Slender!

**The Plan: First, wean them off sweets.
Then gradually cut out fast foods.**

Our children are sick! 76% of all Americans are now overweight; including children. The main culprit is sugar and the deadly combination of SUGAR - SALT - FAT
Read these startling facts:
Since the 1980's the chance of a young adult getting stomach cancer has gone up 70%. Children aged 8-17 are now getting hypertension and diabetes. Children in the 5th grade have elevated cholesterol levels. More than 10% of children and teens have high cholesterol! Chronic illness is spiking among our kids. Guidelines from a leading pediatrics group now advise screening for **high cholesterol prior to puberty.**
New regulations are beginning to call for Mental Health Checks in grade school because their brains are becoming compromised.
I'm serious! I am looking at the studies as I type this!

Beware of the Sugar-Salt-Fat combination found at fast food restaurants. Sugar is purposely added to the foods to create an "addiction".
The Sugar/Fat/Salt combination in fast food is addictive because it increases the hedonic value of food; gives us pleasure. Chicken nuggets or tenders are so popular because they are loaded with salty/sweet batter and fat. Researchers have called them UFO's (unidentified fried objects) Your child can become addicted very quickly! The S-F-S ratio is even used on hamburgers. How do they do it? Sugar, fat, salt are either loaded into the meat and bread or layered on top of it, or both! Cheese fries are a high fat food with MORE fat on top of it. The potato breaks down to sugar in body .Once it is fried and layered with cheese, you are eating salt on fat on fat on sugar. Then you add ketchup - more sugar!

WHAT HAPPENS TO A CHILD'S BODY with constant access to sugar + fat / salt + fat / sugar + fat + salt

- Weight gain
- Their bodies find these foods rewarding and they want to go back for more
- Neurons are stimulated. The sweeter, more fatty the food, the more the neurons fire. The more they fire, the more they will consume and they end up not leaving any food on the plate or in the bag
- A very strong emotional response is triggered over time.

I have seen kids, on a limited lunch hour at school, hop into a car, drive 15 miles to a favorite fast food place, grab the food and eat it in the car on the way back without even getting out of the vehicle! They have to have it!

Tell your kids that it is NOT <u>food if it comes in thru the car window!</u> There is even more at work here in getting our kids addicted. Highly palatable foods are hyper-stimulants. They stimulate the brain to get the same cue in the future (when you see an ad, billboard, picture of French fries) The cue can be an ad, a memory, or even a location. This provokes impulsive behavior. CUE=URGE=REWARD It becomes automated. Did you ever start thinking about fast food or even a doughnut "out of the blue?" You imagine the taste, smell, sensation of eating it? You have been cued. Kids can even become anxious & pre-occupied. Satisfying the urge only ingrains the addiction further.

Only 15% of people can withstand these cues. Most cannot. I urge you; <u>do not let your kids continue down this path!</u>

Fast Food also has a very high "energy density"; the amount of calories an item has in relation to its weight. The portion size may look ok but contains too many calories.

On big burger + fries = twice as many calories as same weight of pasta and salad. <u>One single fast food meal often contains enough calories to satisfy the calorie requirements for an entire day!</u>

BEVERAGES

Coffee drinks are another culprit destroying our young people's health: Frappuccino consists of sugar, fat, salt in coffee! Addicted people line up to order them.

Soft drinks are syrup & carbonated tap water and are also addictive. The liver was not designed to process Coca Cola! Do not offer fruit juices.

Compare drinking 3 apples in one minute to eating 3 apples gradually. The fructose in the juice goes right to the liver where it is converted to fat.

Kids can lose weight just by giving up sweet drinks!

WHAT CAN YOU DO?

1. **Make a rule:** <u>We do not eat in the car.</u>

2. **<u>Scare your kids.</u>** I had my son read Fast Food Nation when he was 14 and to this day he refuses to go into a fast food restaurant. Truly, there are some disgusting passages in that book. It worked for our family! He was able to resist peer pressure after reading it, which is really hard to do!

   Studies say that we are the first generation whose kids will die younger than we do! Say to yourself, "Not MY kids!" If you want to read more, grab the book "The End of Overeating" The research will shock you.

3. Give your child less food, but food that is high in protein. You will be surprised at how much less food it takes to satisfy them.

4. Have your kids get their proper sleep! At least 8-10 hours. 10-12 is even better according to the National Sleep Foundation. Their sleep deprived bodies release adrenaline and cortisol that make them hyper and incapable of focusing and also prevent their brains' restore and repair cycle from completing its work.
   The next step...they are given Ritalin!

5. Make yourself the Sleep Sherriff! You are the boss in your own home. Your children need you to set the limits.

6. Pregnant? You can pass your "fatness" on to your unborn child! If the mother has elevated blood sugar, the developing fetal pancreas will over-produce insulin secreting cells. The baby will store more fat and crave more carbs and sugar. A vicious cycle is born. Stop the cycle in your family!

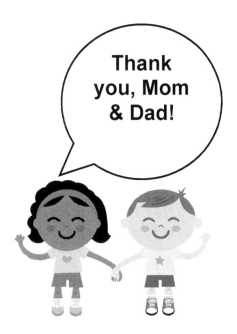

Chapter 19

SUGAR & OTHER MEDICAL CONDITIONS

BRAIN / MOOD

Did you know?

- 30 percent of the calories we take in are used by your BRAIN!
- Sugar and fast-acting processed carbs **disrupt** the brain.
- People with elevated blood sugar levels experience **memory problems**.
- Studies show a link between poor blood sugar control and Alzheimer's!
- **Sugar causes DEPRESSION!** People who eat sugary foods report recurring feelings of despair and hopelessness. The more fast-acting carbs they consume, the more **depressed** they become. Then, the cycle begins whereby the worse they feel, the more they turn to sweets to give them a deceptive, short-lived high. There is a high and chronic level of unhappiness among people who eat too many cakes, cookies, chips, candies, and other quickie carbs. Estimates show that is about 50% of us!
- Sugar causes brain fog, exhaustion and anxiety. You will have no zest, vitality, enthusiasm & optimism with too much sugar. Without it, you will feel HAPPIER & REBORN!

LIBIDO: The News is not good!

Sugar is a libido-quencher/ killer! Sugar-eating people have reported that when they gave in to their sugar cravings, their sex drive "drove off" Why? They have already received a neuro-chemical high from the sweets that they would otherwise have received from sex.

Their desire has been fulfilled and the sugar has now taken precedence over their mate. How sad! Don't deplete your libido. Don't cause marital discord. STAY OFF SUGAR!

WEIGHT LOSS

I have many testimonials from women who have lost weight and dress sizes, as well as men who have lost impressive amounts of weight. One lady called last week to say she lost 12 pounds in one month when she gave up sugar. My husband lost 35 pounds in 5 months, just by eliminating sugars! I myself lost more weight when he went on the program because I became even more vigilant with labels. I did not need to lose weight, but I felt better than ever! A large study showed that eliminating sugar, refined carbs, and also alcohol, for three months, led to weight loss of up to 100 lbs. Seriously! On the other hand, study participants who stepped up their intake of soft drinks and drank one or more per day over the eight years of the study gained, on average, **more than 17 pounds**. Just by drinking an extra soft drink. Take the sugar challenge. I guarantee that you will lose weight!

PMS

More than 74 percent of women have cravings when they are pre-menstrual. During this time the body's pain threshold is reduced so women are predisposed biologically to crave foods that trigger the release of opioids (morphine like substances) that helps them endure cramps and irritability. However, the sugar makes them more edgy or depressed. There are supplements that can do a much better job such as dopamine releasers like L-Tyrosine as well as B-12 and magnesium. Secondly, when we are premenstrual, our serotonin levels drop. Women who feel depressed premenstrually will tend to overeat sweets and other carbs to raise serotonin levels. In other words, we are trying to self-medicate with sugar and carbs. It does not work! It makes you feel worse when your blood sugar subsequently plummets.

Guess what?

The correct types of carbs, such as sweet potatoes, can boost serotonin and reduce PMS symptoms.
Ladies, managing your sugar intake could be one of the most powerful and effective ways to curtail PMS-triggered symptoms.

PERI-MENOPAUSE / MENOPAUSE

During this time estrogen and progesterone levels begin to drop either rapidly, slowly, or erratically. And, because these hormones influence a woman's response to insulin, the shift can affect how sugar is processed by the body. This can lead to rapid weight gain. When you stay off sugar you become less reactive to the hormone changes and have more control over your weight, hot flashes, night sweats, and insomnia!

YEAST

Yeast is caused by the overgrowth of a fungus called *Candida albicans.*

Yeast thrives on sugar. Anything that increases your blood sugar or changes the hormonal balance that regulates blood sugar can cause yeast to grow out of control. A low-sugar diet is your best defense against Candida. If you keep feeding yeast cells they will multiply, and even the best anti-microbial herbs won't keep them in check. Eat a low or no-sugar diet for at least 3 months and your symptoms should disappear. But don't revert to old habits, or the Candida symptoms will quickly return. But you will feel so wonderful; you will not want to revert. I can look at a slice of chocolate cake (my favorite in the past) or boysenberry pie and **just say no!** No sugar drug for me!

By the way, Candida is linked to Fibromyalgia and Chronic Fatigue, so if you suffer from those, stay off sugar!!

PCOS (Polycystic Ovary Syndrome)

High insulin can overwhelm a woman's ovaries to the point where she stops producing progesterone. Instead of progesterone, the ovaries begin to turn out excessive amounts of androgens or "masculine hormones." Androgens and insulin block the development and monthly release of an egg resulting in polycystic ovary syndrome (PCOS), affecting about 10% of women of childbearing age. It is a leading cause of infertility. PCOS is characterized by high or normal estrogen levels high androgens, and low progesterone. Symptoms of the condition are obesity, especially middle-of-the-body obesity, acne, oily skin, facial and breast hair and head hair loss.

A woman may not ovulate for months at a time and then have a very heavy period. When you create an insulin imbalance your reproductive system can shut down completely. People, it is a simple fact: Sick people don't reproduce!

Committing to a diet of no sugar or quickie carbs is one of the most important changes for a woman with PCOS.

Also, it is extremely beneficial to bring progesterone into balance and for this you use physiologic doses of progesterone.

For severe cases, your doctor may recommend:
- Spironolactone, which blocks androgen action at the cell level.
- Metformin, a drug that sensitizes the body to insulin and allows the insulin levels to go down.

In my opinion, it is best to use drugs for a limited amount of time and try to use more natural methods.

WRINKLES
Low Sugar = Fewer Wrinkles
Sugar is very damaging to the skin because sugar molecules attach to collagen fibers, causing them to become stiff and inflexible. This leads to wrinkling, a leathery look, and loss 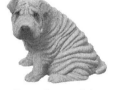 of elasticity of your skin. Glycogen also discolors skin so dark patches may appear. Our bodies are quite miraculous: Collagen can be rebuilt. Stop eating sugar and the free radicals will reduce, and the damage to collagen will reduce.

- If you took some skin cells, put them into a Petri dish, and let them grow, and then added a few drops of sugar, inflammatory chemicals go up by 1,000 percent over the baseline of an hour
- "Anything that has a beneficial effect on the brain makes the skin look better", Dr. Perricone says. If sugar is bad for the brain, then it is **horrible** for the skin.
- Scientists also say that skin tags, those little flaps of skin that crop up in the armpit, neck, or groin area are "external symptoms of insulin resistance."

CANCER

Researchers in British Columbia compared the effects of a low-carb diet to a typical "Western" diet (high in carbs and low in protein). Both groups were fed equal calories.

They found that **carcinogens grew slower in the low carb/high protein diet**. Mice who had been genetically predisposed to develop breast cancer and ate the high carb diet had rates of cancer nearly 50% by the age of one year, whereas NO TUMORS WERE DETECTED in the mice fed the low carb diet.

Sugar feeds tumors!
Protect yourself against cancer
by staying off sugar!

Yummy Italian Spaghetti Squash (Con't)

Remove seeds from cooked squash. Scoop squash from shell with a fork into individual bowls separating strands.

Top with sauce, garnish with fresh basil and sprinkle with parmesan cheese.

Notes:
For protein I like:
Pre-cooked:
Sliced chicken breast
Turkey sausage whole or sliced
Turkey or beef meatballs

If you want to spend the extra time, you can make a nice Bolognese sauce by sautéing:
1 pound ground turkey or beef with Italian spices, salt & pepper,

Add to sauce and simmer 45 minutes

You have your favorite spaghetti topping recipes. The squash will love them all.

The secret is you are no longer eating white pasta.
You are going you LOVE the substitution.

Spaghetti Squash Greek Style

Ingredients:
- 1 squash
- 2 TBS. olive oil
- 1 onions, chopped
- 2 cloves garlic minced
- 2 cups chopped fresh tomatoes, grape or cherry tomatoes are great
- 1 cup diced tomatoes, drained
- ½ cup crumbled or chopped feta cheese
- 10 sliced black olives (Kalamata are the best)
- Fresh herbs of your choice or 1 TBS of Greek seasoning

Directions:

Pierce skin of squash with knife in about 4 places. Then, microwave on high for 7 minutes.

Remove, cut in half, and place cut-side down in oval dish with ¼ inch of water. Microwave on high another 5 minutes until flesh is tender. Time may vary.

Heat oil, sauté onion till tender
Add garlic; cook 3 – 4 minutes. Mix in tomatoes and olives. Add fresh herbs like parsley, oregano.

Scoop squash from shell & separate into strands. Toss with tomato mixture. Top with fresh herbs and Feta cheese.

Optional: You can sauté other vegetables with the onion. I like red & green peppers.

YUM!

Chicken, Kale & White Bean Soup

Ingredients:
- 1 pack of pre-cooked chicken breast
- 1 ½ TBS olive oil
- 2 cloves chopped garlic
- 1 medium – large onion, chopped
- 2 medium carrots, sliced
- 1 can (15 ounces) cannellini beans, drained
- 4 cups chicken stock
- 1–2 pounds kale, chopped (or other greens like spinach, collard greens. Trader Joe's makes a nice mix
- 1 leek, chopped
- Salt & pepper to taste
- 1 TB Bouquet garnie spice
- 1 Tsp. Italian spice

Directions:

In a large pot heat oil, sauté garlic, carrot, leek & onion 5 – 7 minutes

Mash ½ can of beans with fork or potato masher, add to onion & garlic mix.

Add chicken broth and bring to boil.
Add seasonings and chopped kale. Kale will entirely fill pot, but will cook down.

Simmer 20 minutes.

Add chicken and remaining beans then simmer 10 minutes more.

Chicken, Kale & White Bean Soup (con't)

Serve with fresh grated parmesan cheese. Fantastic!

Notes:
You can also use any pre-cooked chicken or turkey sausage. There are some great flavors like chicken jalapeno or chicken with sundried tomato and basil.

I also like to put some red pepper flakes in my bowl! Let's get the metabolism going!

Skinny Mashed Potatoes

Ingredients:
- 4 cups cauliflower florets (This is 1 medium head of cauliflower)
- 3 Tablespoons milk, heated
- 1 tablespoon butter

Directions:

Steam or microwave cauliflower until tender.
Drain cauliflower so it is really dry.

Puree in food processer or just mash with potato masher.
I like using a potato masher because I like this dish more chunky.

Add milk, butter, sea salt and pepper. Mix well.
Top with chives or whatever you usually do with mashed potatoes.

Option: Add garlic powder & rosemary.

Another option "Fried Skinny Potatoes":
Put a little olive oil in a skillet, add steamed cauliflower, add some Italian spices and sauté it for about 5 – 7 minutes. My husband's favorite!

Baked Asparagus

Ingredients:
- 1 bunch asparagus
- 1 TB olive oil
- Sea salt & garlic powder to taste

Directions:

Place asparagus in baking pan or cooking sheet with sides

Spray or brush with olive oil and sprinkle with sea salt and garlic powder.

Squeeze lemon over finished product.

Roasted Veggie Combo

This recipe will change your relationship
with veggies!

Put a combo of any of the following in a big metal roasting pan. The smaller you cut the pieces, the browner and sweeter the veggies will get.

Ingredients:
- Cauliflower
- Onions (red or yellow) – the more the merrier because they help carmelization
- Carrots
- Red bell peppers
- Yams
- Pea pods
- Zucchini
- Turnips
- Brussel sprouts
- Beets
- Broccoli

In other words, just grab what you think looks good in your market.

Directions:
Cut the vegetables into a size you like. (Smaller size will cook more quickly).

Lay the vegetables out in a single layer – they will caramelize better and taste sweeter.
Drizzle with olive oil. Add sea salt, pepper & your favorite spices. Rosemary and oregano are great!

Bake at 425° for 30-40 minutes.

Roasted Veggie Combo (Con't)

For browner veggies, bake at 450°.

Veggies will have some brown edges when done. You can also drizzle with Balsamic when done.

YUM! Also, left-overs make a great snack!

So-Easy Baked Chicken

These chicken breasts are SO tasty. Make extras and use for breakfast or lunches.
Pair with Skinny mashed "potatoes" and baked asparagus for dinner.

Ingredients:
- 4 – 6 chicken breasts with ribs
- Sea salt
- Your favorite seasonings*
- Paprika

Directions:

Place breasts in roasting pan.

Lift skin and put your favorite seasoning underneath the skin next to the breast meat.

Shake paprika & sea salt on breast skin. Paprika gives the chicken a beautiful, golden finish.

Bake uncovered 375° for 45 minutes exactly.

Cooked breasts will be nicely browned, moist and succulent.

*Note: Trader Joe's has a great product called   21 Seasoning Sauté that I love OR use any combo of seasonings. Don't be shy!

Stove Top Low-Carb Lasagna

Ingredients:
- 1 TBS olive oil
- 1 pound ground beef or turkey
- 1 medium onion
- 2-4 cloves of garlic
- 1 zucchini, chopped (optional)
- ¼ - ½ cup of Ricotta cheese
- Italian seasoning
- Low-fat mozzarella cheese
- 1 cup favorite spaghetti sauce (Can use more as desired if you like a "wetter" lasagna
- Sea salt
- Fresh ground pepper

Direction:

In a skillet, sauté onion & garlic in olive oil.

Add ground meat and zucchini, sea salt & pepper and sauté until meat is cooked.

Add spaghetti sauce and cook 10 minutes.

Add Ricotta cheese and any additional Italian spice to taste. Stir to blend and simmer until cheese is heated through.

Add mozzarella at end and stir till heated.
Add basil, stir and serve.

Eat to your hearts content!

Once you get the hang of it, you can make this recipe in a jiffy.

Hoffman Holiday Frittata

I make this recipe on holidays when I want my family to have a fun, high protein, fulfilling breakfast prior to any festivities. Easy, delicious, and pretty for company

Ingredients:
- 6 liquid egg whites or 6 separated egg whites
- 6 mushrooms, sliced
- 1 onion
- 1 red pepper
- ¼ cup broccoli florets, cut small
- 1 cup of spinach (optional)
- Any other veggies. I like asparagus & cauliflower
- 2 TBS olive oil
- Fresh or dried herbs of your choice. I like Italian seasoning
- 1–2 slices of Swiss cheese, sliced into thin strips

Directions:

Add olive oil to non-stick skillet and heat on medium – high heat.

Add onion and sauté for 3 minutes. Add all other veggies and cook until golden brown & tender.

Whisk egg whites with 2 tablespoons of parmesan cheese, herbs, sea salt and cracked black pepper

Pour egg mixture into pan and with a spatula, move mixture from side to side so it seeps under the veggies.

Hoffman Holiday Frittata (con't)

Eggs will start to solidify and crust will begin to form at your edges.
Continue to coax liquid egg mix to bottom of pan.

When eggs begin to appear almost set, lay slices of Swiss cheese on top and let it melt.

Remove pan from stove top and put under broiler for about 3 minutes until top is golden brown.

Wait about 3 minutes and slice into pie-shaped wedges.

Serve with fresh fruit salad or sliced strawberries. Have a bowl of salsa on hand and some hot sauce.

Note: To use fresh eggs, just separate them and use only the whites OR use ½ of the yolks and all the whites.

You can use virtually ANY veggies in a frittata and any cheese.

Great left-over too!

Heavenly Chicken Stir Fry

Ingredients:
- 3 TBS oil
- Pre-cooked boneless chicken strips, left over steak or pork, cut into strips
- ¼ cup low-salt soy sauce
  OR 1/8 cup soy sauce & 1/8 cup sherry
- Your choice of veggies OR purchase a bag of prepared stir fry mix (easiest!)
- 1 TB fresh garlic, minced
- 1 TB fresh ginger, grated or sliced thin
- ¼ cup of peanuts or cashews, optional

Directions:

Pre-marinate your protein in ¼ cup low-salt soy sauce or 1/8 cup soy sauce & 1/8 cup sherry
Doesn't need to marinate long; 10 minutes is fine.

Cut your own veggies if you are using your own
I use: Onions, shredded carrots, snow pea pods, yellow squash, scallions, broccoli crowns, or shredded cabbage.

Note: You can add water chestnuts, cherry tomatoes (halved), asparagus, or spinach. Be creative!

Add 1 tablespoon oil to a pan and stir fry your protein 2 – 3 minutes then remove protein from pan.

Add 2 tablespoons of oil to pan. Add onion, garlic & ginger and stir fry for 1 minute.
Add other veggies, stir fry for about 4–5 minutes.

Return protein to pan.

Heavenly Chicken Stir Fry (continued)

You can now throw in the peanuts or cashews.

Stir in your favorite Asian sauce to desired wetness. (I prefer my stir fry on the dry side)
You can make your own sauce or buy one at the grocery store. Some of the Asian sauces you find in grocery stores are too thick, so I dilute them with chicken broth.

Here is *my favorite* sauce:
- ¼ cup chicken broth
- ¼ cup soy sauce
- 2 teaspoons rice vinegar
- 2 teaspoons sesame oil
- Shake of red pepper flakes

Turkey Meatballs

Ingredients:
- 1 pound ground turkey
- 3 – 5 garlic cloves, minced
- ½ cups finely chopped parsley
- 2 eggs
- ½ cups milk
- ½ cup grated cheese
- ¾ cups Italian bread crumbs
- 1 TBS olive oil
- 1 onion, minced finely
- 1 Tsp. sea salt
- ½ Tsp. cracked black pepper

Directions:

Place all ingredients in large bowl and mix thoroughly. Let stand half an hour.

Note: You can add any other seasonings of your choice. For example, 1 Tsp. Italian spice.
Shape into medium size meatballs.
Makes about 12 meat balls.

Place on cookie sheet and bake at 350 degrees for 30-35 minutes until meatballs look slightly browned.

My favorite snack! These freeze really well!

Don't worry! – That ¾ cup of bread crumbs "binds" the meat balls and won't spike your insulin.

Cauliflower Pizza Crust

Wow! This is an incredible discovery. Please try it at least once.

Ingredients:
4 cups cauliflower rice, steamed & strained (1 head = 4 cups)
1 egg, beaten
1/3 cup soft goat cheese (called chevre)
1 ½ tsp dried oregano or Italian Spice Mix
Pinch of salt

Step 1: Pulse batches of raw cauliflower florets in a food processor, until a rice-like texture is achieved. It actually will look like rice.

Step 2: Fill a large pot with about an inch of water, and bring it to a boil. Turn off heat. Add the "rice" and cover; let it steam for 5 minutes. Drain into a fine-mesh strainer. Once you've strained the rice, transfer it to a clean, thin dishtowel. Wrap up the steamed rice in the dishtowel, twist and squeeze the excess moisture out. Get it as dry as you can.

Step 3: Shape the dough. In a large bowl, mix strained rice, beaten egg, goat cheese, and spices. Use your hands and mix it really well. Press the dough out onto a baking sheet lined with parchment paper, or use a pizza stone. Keep the dough about 1/3 inch thick. Make the edges a little higher for a crust effect.

Step 4: Bake for 35-40 minutes at 400°F
The crust will be firm, and golden brown when finished.

Add any toppings and return to oven. Bake for 5 – 10 more minutes

Cauliflower Pizza Crust (Con't)

Marguerite Topping
Drizzle olive oil over crust and spread with brush.
I used an olive mister.
Apply:
- A thin layer of tomato sauce
- A thin layer of mozzarella
- Garlic powder
- Thinly sliced tomatoes sprinkled with sea salt.
- Add 4 basil leaves cut into strips.

Cook in oven 5 – 10 more minutes
Sprinkle with parmesan cheese and serve.

My office ate the entire pie and LOVED it.
So tasty!

Chapter 21

Conclusion

Try a week of just protein, or even a few days.
Go slow but steady.

ACCOUNTABILITY WORKS!
Studies show that this is true! I have heard journaling recommended because the journalists lost 3 times as much weight. I have a better idea: Take photos of your meals/snacks and share them with an encouraging friend OR send them to my Facebook page and I will help you. You only need 5 sessions to make something stick as a habit. Make this competitive. We all LOVE a game!

Patience please....you are improving your health, blood pressure, cholesterol.
It may have taken years for you to get to this point. Every step in the right direction will make you feel better. A body clear of excess sugars and carbs will begin to feel GREAT in terms of energy, mood, sleep, and libido as well as losing weight. DO NOT obsess over ONE meal! This is your new journey and the road may meander, but you will get back on track!

You will also begin to notice that sugary things begin to taste WAY TOO SWEET after you have weaned yourself I used to LOVE pie, but today I cannot find any slice of pie that is not too sweet for me to enjoy. It will happen for you, too. Remember that sugar is addictive, so you may need some 5-HTP, L-Tyrosine or GABA to help you out.

YOU WILL NOT BE STARVNG YOURSELF!
You can eat a lot of food if you give up the empty carbs.
Do not consider this a diet. We do not want to use words
with "die" in them!

THE GOOD NEWS:
Once you start eliminating the "bad" carbs you will find:
- You do not think about food as much as you used to....only when you are hungry
- You will feel more energetic
- You may not need to snack as much, although I do encourage healthy snacks
- Your mood will be more even as blood sugar remains stable (There is a great product for keeping blood sugar stable called PGX. I LOVE it! Call me if you would like a sample. You put it in yogurt or any other moist food. It helps you to burn fat for fuel and lose weight. It also creates a feeling of satiety while you are changing to your new lifestyle.
- Blood pressure should come down as the kidneys excrete the sodium they have retained due to high insulin levels
- YOU WILL LEAD A LONGER & HEALTHIER LIFE

> "For I know the plans I have for YOU, declares the Lord" Jeremiah 29:11
> I want you HEALTHY to fulfill those plans.
> Call me if you need a Cheerleader or a Diet Buddy! 877 539-6200

CONGRATULATIONS!

YOU ARE NOW ON YOUR WAY TO BALANCING YOUR WEIGHT and going back to being "you" again!

The process of change is mostly mental. Actual eating is a detail. Eating habits that lower weight are actually NORMAL eating habits...You need an emotional change, not a diet drug or surgery.

You finally will be able to look forward to a food "treat" without feeling a physical or emotional charge. I am so excited for you to achieve your new mood balance and control over what and when you eat!

Trust me, this plan works! I would love to hear from you at any time before, during, or after your Good Mood Diet Plan! **Please let me know of your progress. I want to help you!**

It is my mission to get 1 million people and their families to shed their belly fat, feel like themselves again and prevent diseases like type 2 diabetes and heart disease and obesity by eating delicious, healthy food. THEN, I will go on to the NEXT million people. I need your help!

In the meantime, know that in God's eyes,
"Every Body is a Good Body"
With love,
Barbara Hoffman

"Oh, taste and see that the Lord is good!" Psalm 34:8
"How sweet are your words to my taste, sweeter than honey to my mouth!" Psalm 119:103

Dear Friends,

I sincerely hope that you enjoyed this book and that you will join me in my mission to turn the tides of the obesity epidemic. Please keep in touch, I am constantly updating my information. There is so much to learn (and sometimes unlearn) about our optimal health and well-being. I believe if we stick together, we have the best chance for making this a healthier world for all families.

I would LOVE to hear from you, too! I am collecting material all the time to add to my research, and I want to hear your success story!

Do you have a question that was not answered?
Do you have a testimony that will help other women?
Do you have a comment or observation?
Or would you like to be on my mailing list?

You can contact me at any of my websites:
www.bhnformulas.com
www.2prn.com
www.askbarbarahoffman.com
www.newhealthyskin.com

You may write to me at:

Barbara Hoffman
P.O. Box 1292
Corona del Mar, CA   92625

Email me at barbara@askbarbarahoffman.com

If you would like to call me or fax, the numbers are:

Phone: (877) 880-0170
Fax: (800) 618-1314

May you be blessed and be in good health all the days of your life!

With love,
Barbara Hoffman

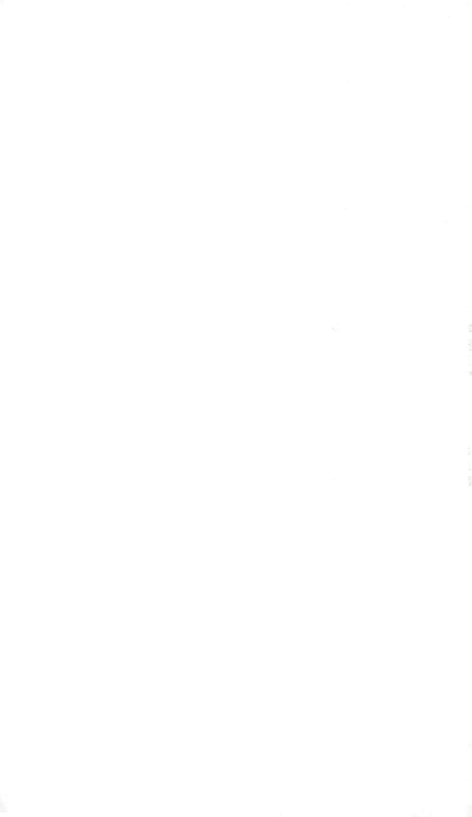

supplements

folic acid

L- Tyrosine

phosphatidylserene

(see Bottom of page 61

free Booklet — "natural
progesterone for you"

Made in the USA
Columbia, SC
03 April 2023

14731251R00083